Naturopathy

Medicinal Plants for Herbal Healing

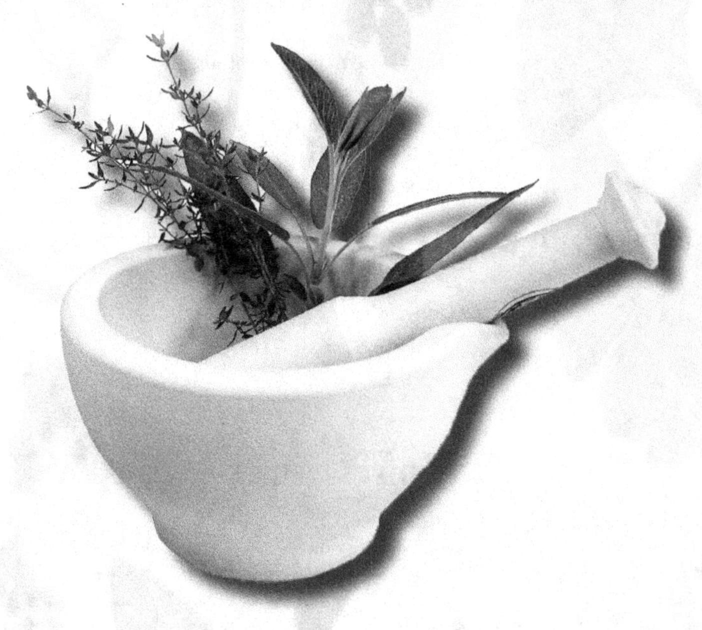

V&S PUBLISHERS

Published by:

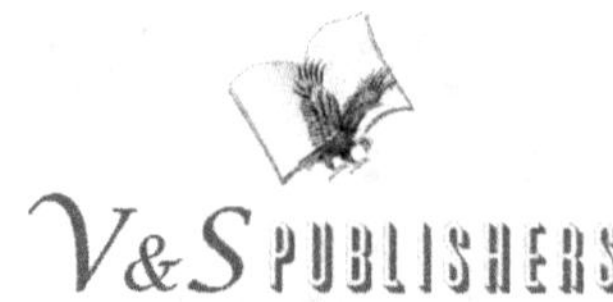

V&S PUBLISHERS

F-2/16, Ansari road, Daryaganj, New Delhi-110002
☎ 23240026, 23240027 • *Fax:* 011-23240028
Email: info@vspublishers.com • *Website:* www.vspublishers.com

Regional Office : Hyderabad
5-1-707/1, Brij Bhawan (Beside Central Bank of India Lane)
Bank Street, Koti, Hyderabad - 500 095
☎ 040-24737290
E-mail: vspublishershyd@gmail.com

Branch Office : Mumbai
Jaywant Industrial Estate, 1st Floor–108, Tardeo Road
Opposite Sobo Central Mall, Mumbai – 400 034
☎ 022-23510736
E-mail: vspublishersmum@gmail.com

BUY OUR BOOKS FROM: AMAZON FLIPKART

© **Copyright:** *V&S* PUBLISHERS
ISBN 978-93-505718-5-9
Edition 2020

Publisher's Note

Medicinal Plants and Herbs have been used by mankind from times immemorial, particularly in the traditional Indian systems of medicine, such as *Ayurveda* and *Homeopathy*. Some of them are even toxic, but of immense pharmaceutical value.

Basically, plants have the ability to synthesise a wide variety of chemical compounds that are used to perform important biological functions and to defend against attack from predators, like insects, fungi, bacteria and viruses, thus, protecting us from a number of deadly diseases like Cancer, Tuberculosis, AIDS and many incurable Skin and Venereal diseases.

The study of plants for medicinal purposes is called as *Herbalism* or *Herbal Medicine* and the usage of these medicinal plants for treatment and cure of different types of diseases is known as **Naturopathy**. This book contains an *exhaustive list of about 200 medicinal plants and herbs* which are used totally or in parts, such as their roots, stems, leaves, or barks, crushed or decocted, boiled or mixed with water or honey, etc., to treat innumerable commonly occurring diseases like: cough and cold, fevers, pneumonia, skin diseases, indigestion, diarrhoea, asthma, and even snake-bites and scorpion-stings.

Though all the usage and treatments suggested in the book have been authenticated by the author, yet a doctor's advice is a must before consuming or applying these plant extracts on your body.

All said and done, the book has been aimed to enlighten all its readers about the *Natural Cure and Healing of several diseases with Plants and Plant Products, which generally do not have any side effects and help to completely eradicate the diseases from their roots*. Hope the book is beneficial to all and serves its purpose well. We would be glad to receive your valuable suggestions and queries on the subject to make it all the more appealing and worth reading..............

Contents

Publisher's Note		3
1.	Kariyat	6
2.	Hophead	7
3.	Porcupine Flower	8
4.	Bell Weed	9
5.	Blue Fox Tail	10
6.	Marsh Barbel	11
7.	Malabar Nut	12
8.	Gandarusa	13
9.	Water Willow	14
10.	Crested Lepidagathis	15
11.	Magenta Plant	16
12.	Nongmangkha	17
13.	Snake Jasmine	18
14.	Karvy	19
15.	Singkrang	20
16.	Sage Leaved Alangium	21
17.	Chives	22
18.	Himalayan Onion	23
19.	Prickly Chaff Flower	24
20.	Two-toothed Chaff Flower	25
21.	Mountain Knot Grass	26
22.	Sessile Joyweed	27
23.	Milk and Wine Lily	28
24.	Marking Nut	29
25.	Sugar Apple	30
26.	Himalayan Thorowax	31
27.	Indian Pennywort	32
28.	Himalayan Hogweed	33
29.	Nepal Hogweed	34
30.	Wild Carrot	35
31.	Batino	36
32.	Sea Mango	37
33.	Indrajao	38
34.	Shrub Vinca	39
35.	Sarpagandha	40
36.	Wild Snake Root	41
37.	Nag Kuda	42
38.	Sweet Indrajao	43
39.	Cabbage Palm	44
40.	Green Milkweed Creeper	45
41.	Gurmar	46
42.	Indian Sarsaparilla	47
43.	Holostemma Creeper	48
44.	Pergularia	49
45.	Indian Ipecac	50
46.	Aloe Vera	51
47.	Common Yarrow	52
48.	Toothache Plant	53
49.	Sticky Daisy	54
50.	Goat Weed	55
51.	Indian Wormwood	56
52.	Spanish Needles	57
53.	Kakronda	58
54.	Safflower	59
55.	Siam Weed	60
56.	Chicory	61
57.	Wild Cosmos	62
58.	Thickhead	63
59.	False Daisy	64
60.	Elephant Foot	65
61.	Burma Agrimony	66
62.	Quick Weed	67
63.	Madras Carpet	68
64.	Hill Gynura	69
65.	Stem Clasping Ligularia	70
66.	Costus	71
67.	Kasturi Kamal	72
68.	Brahma Kamal	73
69.	Snow Lotus	74
70.	St. Paul's Wort	75
71.	Prickly Sow-Thistle	76
72.	Sow Thistle	77
73.	East Indian Globe Thistle	78

74.	Feverfew	79
75.	Giant Mexican Sunflower	80
76.	Little Ironweed	81
77.	Chinese Wedelia	82
78.	Yellow Dots	83
79.	East Himalayan Balsam	84
80.	Chitra	85
81.	Indian Barberry	86
82.	Nepal Mahonia	87
83.	Calabash Tree	88
84.	Katsagon	89
85.	Sausage Tree	90
86.	Roheda	91
87.	Comfrey	92
88.	Indian Borage	93
89.	Shepherd's Purse	94
90.	Indian Olibanum	95
91.	Hatchet Cactus	96
92.	Fever Nut	97
93.	Amaltas	98
94.	Coffee Senna	99
95.	Sita Ashok	100
96.	Tanner's Cassia	101
97.	Asian Spider Flower	102
98.	Garlic Pear Tree	103
99.	Nag Kesar	104
100.	Arjun Tree	105
101.	Baheda	106
102.	Chebulic Myrobalan	107
103.	Grass of the Dew	108
104.	Rudravanti	109
105.	Dwarf Morning Glory	110
106.	Giant Potato	111
107.	Kidney Leaf Morning Glory	112
108.	Painted Spiral Ginger	113
109.	Air Plant	114
110.	Chinese Cucumber	115
111.	Wild Cucumber	116
112.	Umbrella Sedge	117
113.	Karmal	118
114.	Wild Yam	119
115.	Gaub	120
116.	Jamaica Cherry	121
117.	Dwarf Rhododendron	122
118.	Pink Scaly Rhododendron	123
119.	Yellow Scaly Rhododendron	124
120.	Red Physic Nut	125
121.	Graceful Sandmat	126
122.	Suryavarti	127
123.	Triangular Spurge	128
124.	Asthma Weed	129
125.	Willow-Leaved Water Croton	130
126.	Bellyache Bush	131
127.	Kamala Tree	132
128.	Castor Bean Plant	133
129.	Red Sandalwood	134
130.	Red Bush Tea	135
131.	Himalayan Milk Vetch	136
132.	Takoli	137
133.	Shisham	138
134.	West Indian Indigo	139
135.	Pongam Tree	140
136.	Velvet Bean	141
137.	Tree Bean	142
138.	Salaparni	143
139.	Indian Kudzu	144
140.	Sensitive Smithia	145
141.	Trefle Gros	146
142.	Wild Indigo	147
143.	Red Clover	148
144.	Coffee Plum	149
145.	Fried Egg Tree	150
146.	Lesser Swertia	151
147.	Panicled Swertia	152
148.	Stone Flower	153
149.	Ceylon Hydrolea	154
150.	Golden Eye Grass	155
151.	Himalayan Bugle	156
152.	Malabar Catmint	157
153.	Shady Calamint	158
154.	White Dead Nettle	159

Kariyat

Botanical Name:

Andrographis paniculata

Family:

Acanthaceae (**Ruellia family**)

Synonyms:

Justicia paniculata

Common Names:

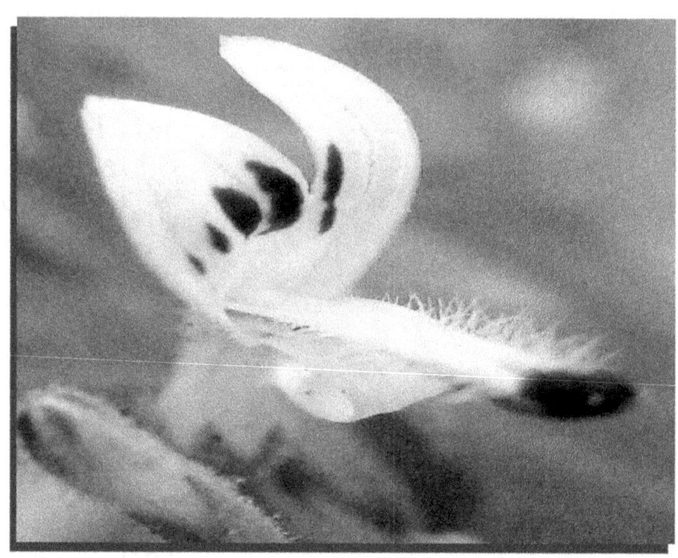

Kariyat, Creat • Hindi: *Kirayat, Kalpanath* • Manipuri: *Vubati* • Marathi: *Oli-kiryata, Kalpa* • Tamil: *Nilavembu* • Malayalam: *Nelavepu, Kiriyattu* • Telugu: *Nilavembu* • Kannada: *Nelaberu* • Bengali: *Kalmegh* • Oriya: *Bhuinimba* • Konkani: *Vhadlem Kiratyem* • Urdu: *Naine-havandi* • Assamese: *Kalmegh* • Gujarati: *Kariyatu* • Sanskrit: *Kalmegha, Bhunimba* • Mizo: *Hnakhapui*

Description:

Kariyat is an erect annual herb extremely bitter in taste in all parts of the plant. It grows erect to a height of 1-4 ft in moist shady places with smooth leaves and white flowers with rose-purple spots on the petals. Stem dark green, 0.3 - 1.0 m in height, 2-6 mm in diameter, quadrangular with longitudinal furrows and wings on the angles of the younger parts, slightly enlarged at the nodes; leaves glabrous, up to 8.0 cm long and 2.5 cm broad, lanceolate, pinnate; flowers small, in lax spreading axillary and terminal racemes or panicles; capsules linear-oblong, acute at both ends, 1.9 cm x 0.3 cm; seeds numerous, sub quadrate, yellowish brown.

Medicinal Uses:

Since ancient times, Kariyat is used as a wonder drug in traditional *Siddha* and *Ayurvedic* systems of medicine as well as in *tribal medicine in India* and some other countries for multiple clinical applications. The therapeutic value of *Kalmegh* is due to its mechanism of action which is perhaps by *enzyme* induction. The plant extract exhibits *antityphoid* and *antifungal* activities.

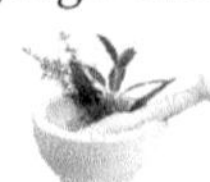

Hophead

Botanical Name:
Barleria lupulina

Family:
Acanthaceae (**Ruellia family**)

Common Names:
Hophead, Philippine Violet • Bengali: *Vishellakarani*

Description:
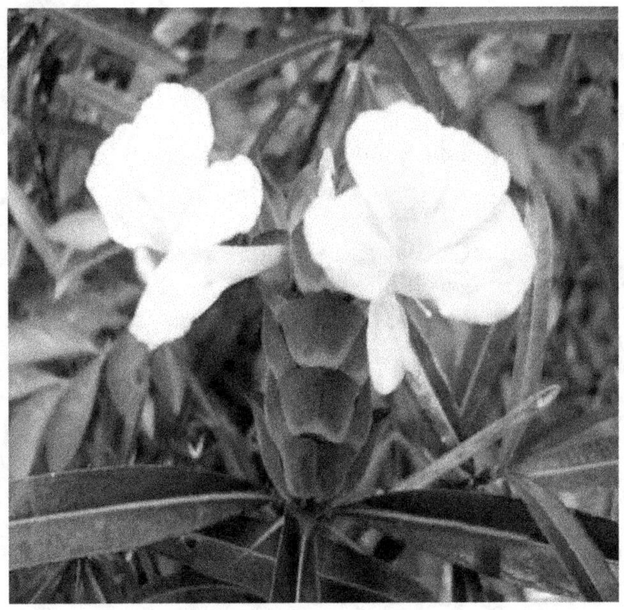

Hophead is a popular medicinal plant distributed in mountains of southern and western India. Shrubbery plant with single dark green leaves, red-brown branches, and flowers that bloom in upright spikes. It is an erect shrub with smooth, hairless stems and leaves. Leaves narrowly obovate, spine-tipped, 3.5-9 cm long, 0.8-1.2 cm wide. Flowers occur in a terminal spike with overlapping bracts which are broadly ovate, 15 mm long, green with purple upper half. Flower consists of a 3m long corolla tube, opening into 1 cm long petals. Longer stamen filaments 2 cm long; shorter stamens fertile. Style is 3 cm long and smooth.

Medicinal Uses:
Traditional and therapeutic use is anti-inflammatory for insect bites, its fresh leaves are used for herpes simplex, and roots for anti-inflammatory centipede bites.

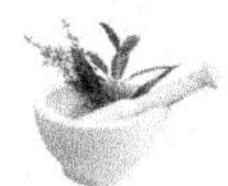

Porcupine Flower

Botanical Name:

Barleria prionitis

Family:

Acanthaceae (**Ruellia family**)

Common Names:

Porcupine flower, Barleria • Hindi: *Vajradanti*
• Tamil: *Kundan* • Kannada: *Mullu goranti*
• Malayalam: *Kuttivetila* • Gujarati:
Pilikantashelio

Description:

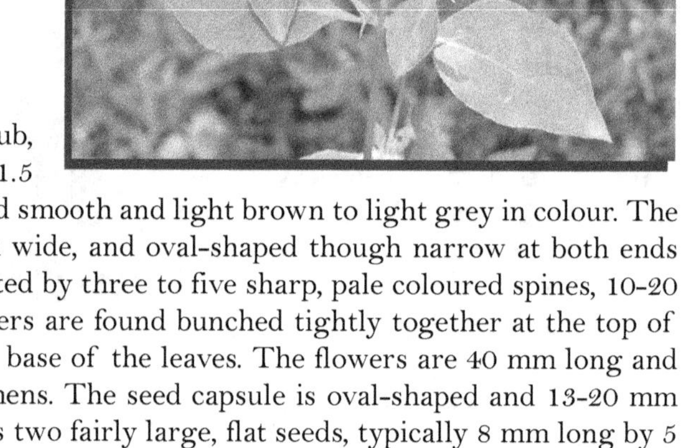

Porcupine flower is an erect, prickly shrub, usually single-stemmed, growing to about 1.5 m tall. The stems and branches are stiff and smooth and light brown to light grey in colour. The leaves are up to 100 mm long and 40 mm wide, and oval-shaped though narrow at both ends (ellipsoid) The base of the leaves is protected by three to five sharp, pale coloured spines, 10-20 mm long. The yellow-orange tubular flowers are found bunched tightly together at the top of the plant, but they also occur singly at the base of the leaves. The flowers are 40 mm long and tubular, with several long protruding stamens. The seed capsule is oval-shaped and 13-20 mm long, with a sharp pointed beak. It contains two fairly large, flat seeds, typically 8 mm long by 5 mm wide, covered with matted hairs. Barleria has a central tap root, with lateral roots branching off in all directions.

Medicinal Uses:

It has numerous medicinal properties including *treating fever, respiratory diseases, toothache, joint pains* and a variety of other ailments; and it has several cosmetic uses. A mouthwash made from root tissue is used to relieve toothache and treat *bleeding gums*. The whole plant, leaves, and roots are used for a variety of purposes in traditional Indian medicine. For example, the leaves are used to promote healing of wounds and to relieve joint pains and toothaches. Because of its antiseptic properties, extracts of the plant are incorporated into herbal cosmetics and hair products to promote skin and scalp health.

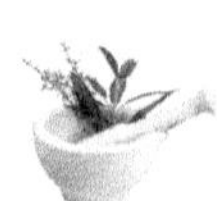

Bell Weed

Botanical Name:
Dipteracanthus prostratus

Family:
Acanthaceae (**Ruellia family**)

Synonyms:
Ruellia prostrata

Common Names:
Bell Weed, Prostrate Wild Petunia, Black weed
• Marathi: Kali dhawani • Tamil: Pottakanchi •
Malayalam: Upudali • Telugu: Neelambaram •
Gujarati: Kalughavani, Kali Dhraman

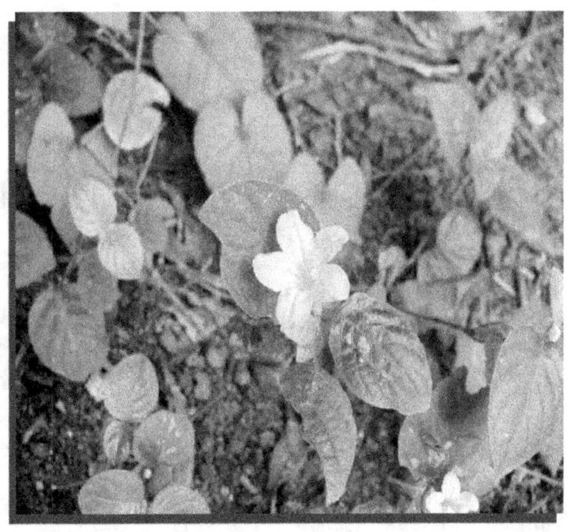

Description:
Bell Weed is a prostrate perennial herb, with stems often rooting at the nodes. Ovate green leaves, 2-10 cm long, have lower surface conspicuously paler. Leaf stalk is 5-30 mm long. Flowers occur solitary in the leaf axils, each one subtended by oblanceolate to ovate bracts 1.5-2.3 cm long. Sepals 5, linear, 6-10 mm long. Flowers are violet blue to occasionally nearly white, 2.4-3.2 cm long, the petals slightly spreading. Capsules are club-shaped, 1.5-2 cm long, densely covered with fine hairs. Flowering: August-September.

Medicinal Uses:
It is believed to be anti-cancer against the epidermis of the nasopharynx region and slightly hypoglycemic.

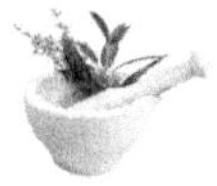

Blue Fox Tail

Botanical Name:
Ecbolium linneanum

Family:
Acanthaceae **(Ruellia family)**

Synonyms:
Justicia ecbolia

Common Names:
Blue Fox Tail, Blue Justicia • Bengali: *Neel Kantha* • Hindi: *Udajati* • Kannada: *Kappubobbuli, Kappukuruni* • Malayalam: *Karinkurinni, Kuranta* • Marathi: *Dhakta adulsa, Ranaboli. Ekboli* • Sanskrit: *Nila-sahacharah* • Tamil: *Nilambari* • Telugu: *Chikatiquratappa, Nakkatoka*

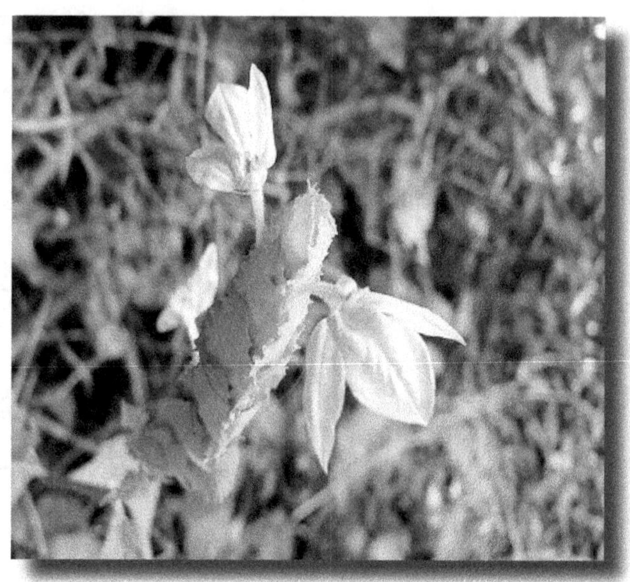

Description:
Blue Fox Tail is a shrubby plant, with four-sided flower-spikes at the end of the branches. Bracts are oval, entire and mucronate. Leaves are elliptic-oblong, narrowed at both ends, and velvety. Flowers are large, greenish blue. The upper lip of the flower is linear, and reflexed. The Blue Fox Tail is found in Mumbai and Konkan regions.

Medicinal Uses:
The plant is used in *gout and dysuria;* decoction of leaves for *stricture.* Roots are given in *jaundice, menorrhagia* and *rheumatism.*

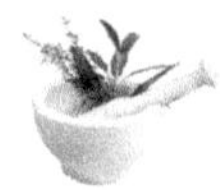

Marsh Barbel

Botanical Name:

Hygrophila schulli

Family:

Acanthaceae (**Ruellia family**)

Synonyms:

Hygrophila auriculata

Common Names:

Marsh Barbel • Hindi: *Gokula kanta* • Marathi: *Talim Khana* • Tamil: *Nirumuli* • Malayalam: *Voyal-chullai* • Telugu: *Kokilakshi* • Kannada: *Kalavankabija* • Bengali: *Shulamardan* • Konkani: *Kalaso* • Sanskrit: *Kokilaksha, Shrinkhali*

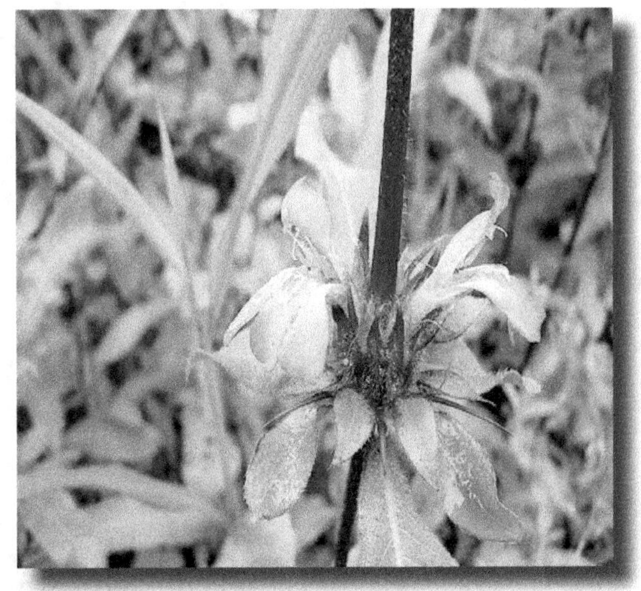

Description:

Marsh Barbel is a stout aquatic perennial herb, 1–2 m high. Erect unbranched stems are hairy near swollen nodes. Densely hairy, lance-like, stalkless leaves, 10–15 cm long, occur in whorls of 6 at each node on the stem. Straight, yellow, 4 cm long spines are present in the axil of each leaf. Flowers occur in 4 pairs at each node. The 3 cm long purple-blue flowers are 2-lipped - the upper lip is 2-lobed and the lower one 3-lobed with lengthwise folds. Flowers open in opposite pairs. Flowering: October–April.

Medicinal Uses:

Kokilaksha, as it is known in Sanskrit, was extensively used in Ayurvedic system of medicine for various ailments like rheumatism, inflammation, jaundice, hepatic obstruction, pain, etc.

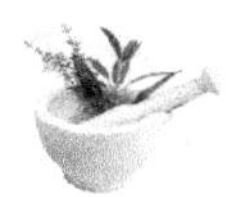

Malabar Nut

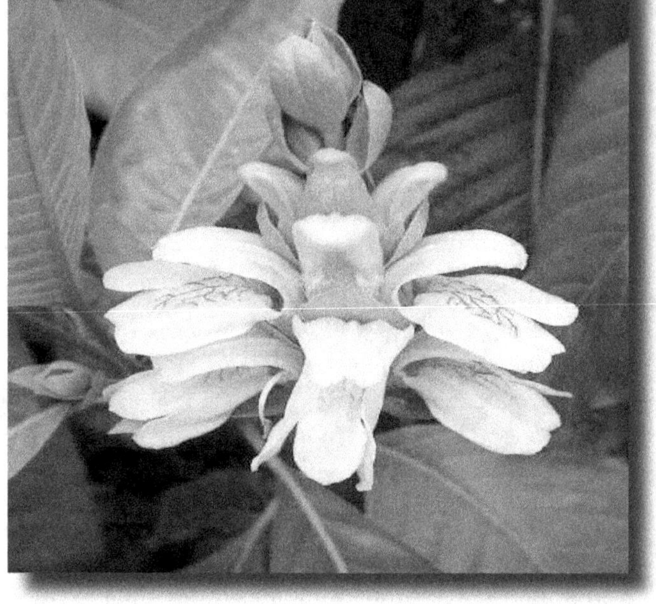

Botanical Name:

Adhatoda vasica

Family:

Acanthaceae (**Ruellia family**)

Synonyms:

Justicia adhatoda

Common Names:

Malabar Nut • Hindi: *Arusa, Vasala* • Manipuri: *Nongmangkha angouba* • Tamil: *Adatodai* • Bengali: *Basak*

Description:

A small evergreen, sub-herbacious bush which grows commonly in open plains, especially in the lower Himalayas. The Leaves are 10 to 16 cms in length, minutely hairy and broadly lanceolate. A herbal plant which requires very little watering and is an extremely hardy plant is Malabar nut. If there is one herbal plant that needs to be singled out for propagation and planting on a large scale, it would be this one. Adhatoda in Tamil, meaning a plant shunned by herbivorous animals. Propagated easily by cuttings, grows to a height of eight to 14 feet and has attractive white flowers.

Medicinal Uses:

Adhatoda is useful for curing coughs, colds and asthma and is easy to administer. It has been used for centuries, and is mentioned in Sanskrit scriptures.

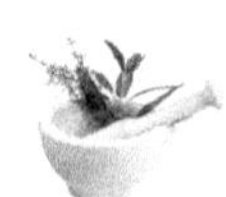

Gandarusa

Botanical Name:

Justicia gendarussa

Family:

Acanthaceae (**Ruellia family**)

Synonyms:

Gendarussa vulgaris, Adhatoda subserrata

Common Names:

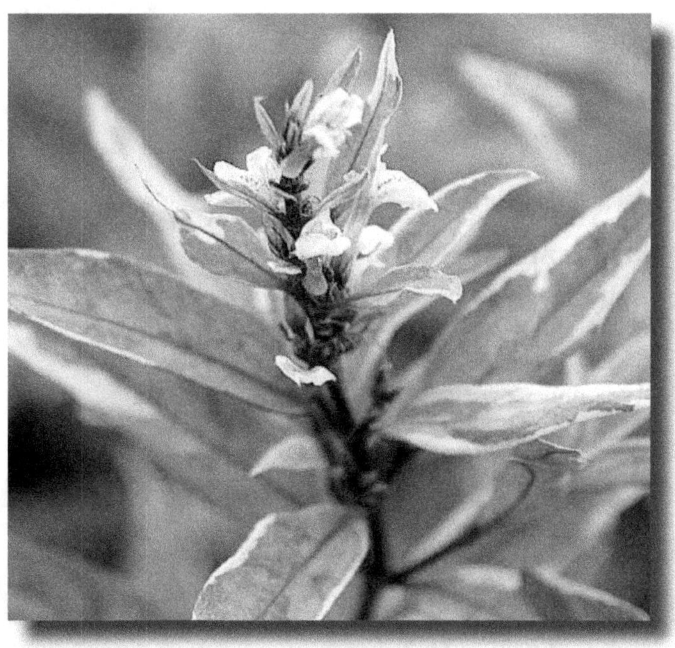

Gandarusa, Warer willow • Hindi: *Nili nargandi, Kala bashimb* • Marathi: *Tev, bakas, Kalaadulsa* • Tamil: *Karunochi, Vadaikkutti* • Malayalam: *Karunochchi, Vada-kodi* • Telugu: *Addasaramu, Gandharasamu, Nalla-noch-chili* • Kannada: *Aduthodagidda, Karalakkigidde, Karinekki* • Bengali: *Jagatmadan* • Oriya: *Nilanirgundi* • Assamese: *Tita-bahak, Bishalya karani* • Sanskrit: *Bhutakeshi, Gandharasa, Indrani, Kapika, Krishnanirgundi*

Description:

Gandarusa is an erect, branched, smooth undershrub about 0.8-1.5 m tall. The leaves are lance-shaped, 7-14 cm long, 1-2.5 cm wide and pointed at the ends. The rather small flowers are borne in 4-12 cm long spikes, at the end of the branches or in leaf axils. The teeth of the sepals cup are smooth, linear and about 3 mm long. The flowers are about 1.5 cm long, white or pink, with purple spots. The capsule is club-shaped, about 12 mm long and smooth.

Medicinal Uses:

Gandarusa is reputed for its beneficial effects in *respiratory disorders* like *cough, cold, bronchitis, throat infections, pulmonary infections* and *allergic disorders* like *bronchial asthma*. It is assumed to possess greater medicinal value to yellow vasa plant or *Adhatoda vasica*.

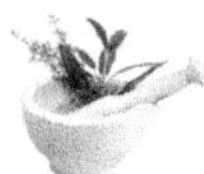

Water Willow

Botanical Name:

Justicia procumbens

Family:

Acanthaceae **(Ruellia family)**

Common Names:

Water Willow • Marathi: *Karambal, Pitpapada, Kalmashi* • Tamil: *Arm, Knteyu, Kotakacalai, Kukkurm* • Konkani: *Ghati Pitpapad*

Description:

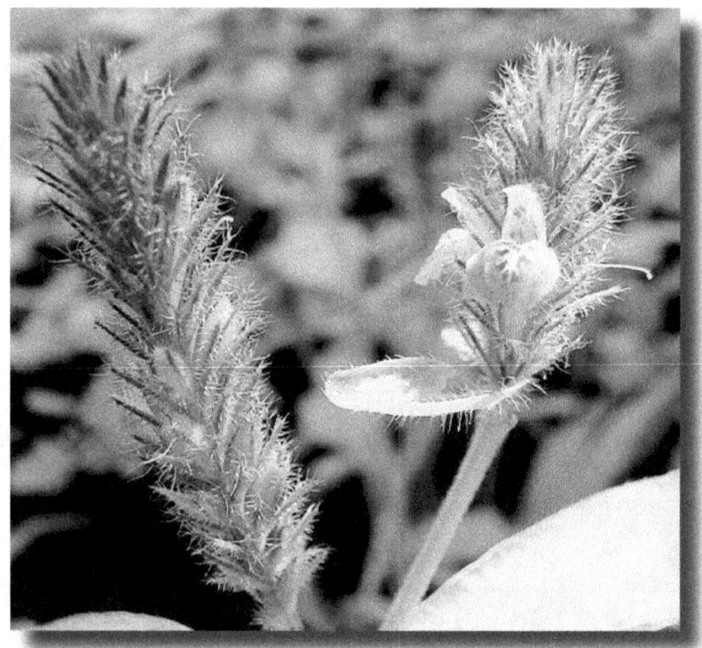

Water Willow is a slender, often tufted, prostrate or ascending, branched perennial herb. The stems are 10–40 cm long. The leaves are elliptic to oblong-ovate or ovate, 7-20 mm long, 5-20 mm wide, obtuse at both ends, and entire or slightly crenate as to margin. The flowers are pink, 6-7 mm long, and borne in terminal, rather dense, cylindric spikes 1-5 cm long and about 5 mm in diameter. The bracts and sepals are green, linear-lanceolate, and hairy. The fruit (capsule) is slightly hairy and about 4 mm long.

Medicinal Uses:

The herb contains a bitter alkaloid taste and that it is used as a substitute for Fumaria. It is alternative and expectorant and is given in the form of *infusion* (1 to 20) in *asthma, coughs* and *rheumatism.* The juice of the leaves is squeezed into the eyes in cases of *ophthalmia.* The odour of the whole plant is unpleasant, and is used in decoction for *backache, plethora* and *flatulence.*

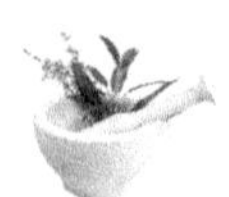

Crested Lepidagathis

Botanical Name:
Lepidagathis cristata

Family:
Acanthaceae **(Ruellia family)**

Common Names:
Crested Lepidagathis • Hindi: *Bukhar Jadi* • Marathi: *Bhui Gend, Bhu terada* • Tamil: *Karappanpoondu* • Kannada: *Surya Kantha*

Description:
Crested Lepidagathis is a perennial herb, with almost no stem. Branches, 20 cm long, arise out of a globose head on the ground, and spread out. Flowers

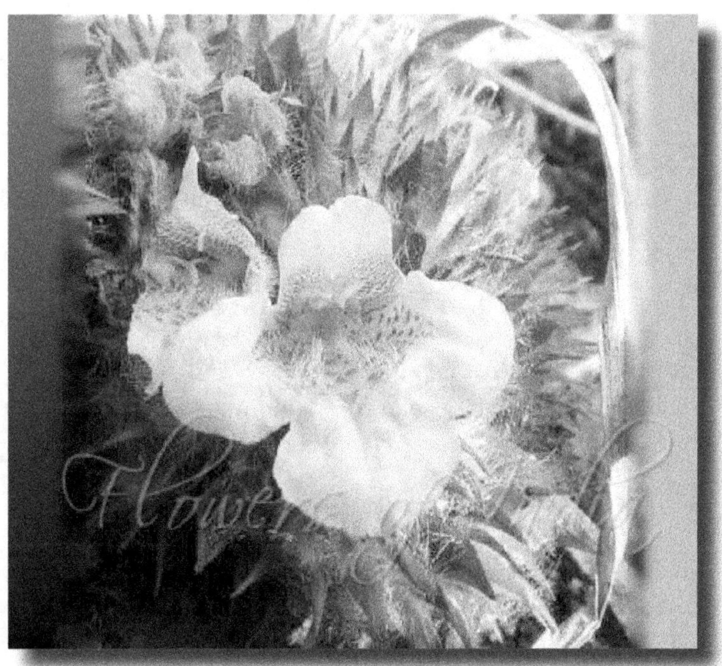

also arise stalkless which are from this globose head. Flowers are pale pink and two-lipped. The upper lip is notched and the lower lip is divided into three lobes.

Medicinal Uses:
In Chattisgarh, they use this herb in treatment of fever, particularly in the treatment of *Malarial fever*. The decoction of leaves is used internally for this purpose. Its utility in treatment of fever has given it the Name *Bukhar Jadi*. In reference literatures, the use of this herb in the treatment of *itchy affections of skin* has been mentioned. The traditional healers of Chhattisgarh Plains are aware of this use. In many parts of Chhattisgarh, the cattle owners use the *decoction of this herb to wash the cattle in rainy* season in order to keep it *free from flies*.

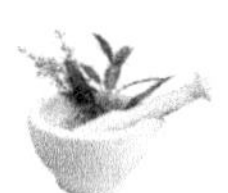

Magenta Plant

Botanical Name:
Peristrophe roxburghiana

Family:
Acanthaceae (**Ruellia family**)

Synonyms:
Peristrophe tinctoria

Common Names:
Peristrophe, Magenta plant • Hindi: Kakajangha

Description:
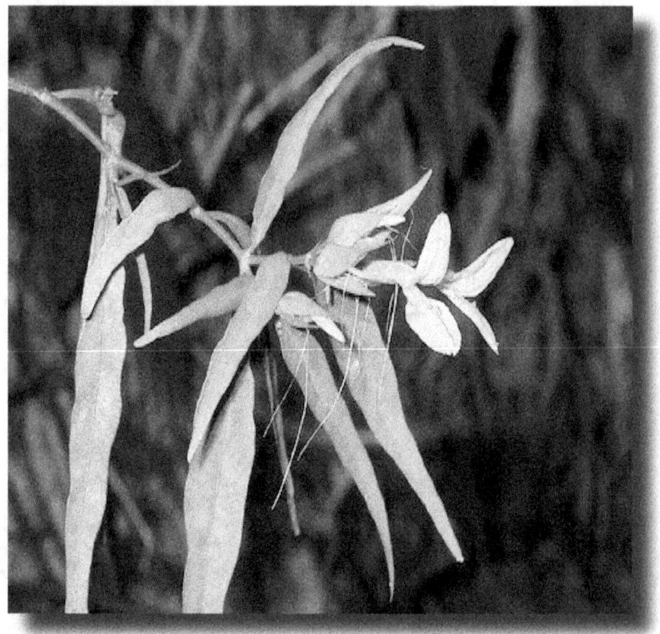

This perennial plant is native to India, and is abundantly found growing in places like Nainital. It is a herb growing up to 50 cm tall. The leaves are lanceolate to ovoid-acute, 2–7.5 cm long and 1–3.5 cm wide. The flowers are two-lobed, the long axis up to 5 cm long, and they are magenta to reddish-violet.

Medicinal Uses:
The plant is used in *traditional Chinese medicine.*

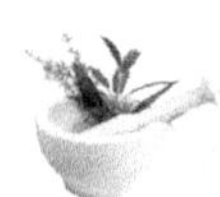

Nongmangkha

Botanical Name:

Phlogacanthus thyrsiformis

Family:

Acanthaceae **(Ruellia family)**

Synonyms:

Phlogacanthus thyrsiflorus, Justicia thyrsiformis, Justicia thyrsiflora

Common Names:

Manipuri: *Nongmangkha* • Assamese: *Banheka*

Description:

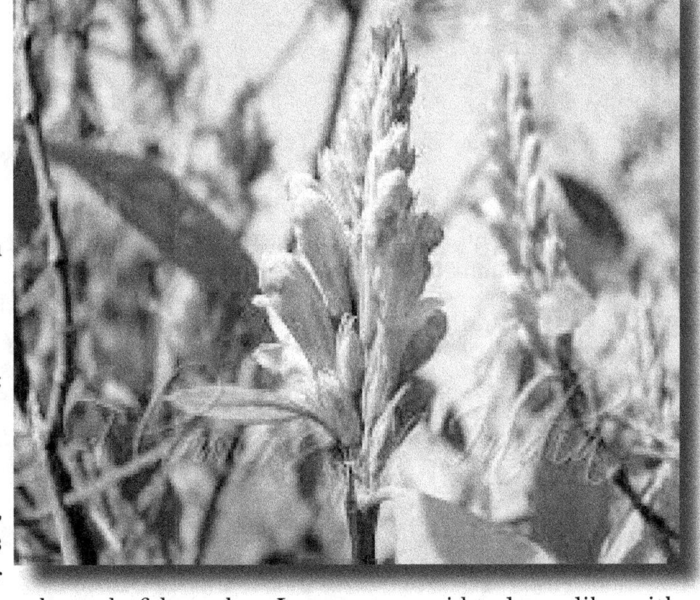

Nongmangkha is a gregarious shrub, common in the Manipur valley. This plant has long orange-red tubular flowers, appearing in upright spikes at the end of branches. Leaves are ovoid to lance-like, with smooth margins. In Manipur, it is an extremely popular medicinal plant.

Medicinal Uses:

In Manipur, local people prefer it to *Malabar* Nut (*Justicia adhatoda*). It is useful for *curing coughs, colds* and *asthma* and is easy to administer. Flowers are *antidote to pox, prevents skin diseases* like *sore, scabies*, etc.

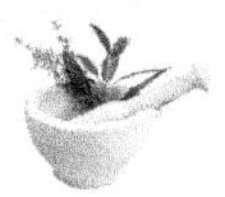

Snake Jasmine

Botanical Name:
Rhinacanthus nasutus

Family:
Acanthaceae (**Ruellia family**)

Synonyms:
Rhinacanthus nasuta, Justicia nasuta, Rhinacanthus communis

Common Names:
Snake Jasmine, Dainty Spurs • Hindi: *Palakjuhi, Juhipani* • Marathi: *Gajkarni* • Tamil: *Uragamalli, Nagamalli* • Malayalam: *Nagamulla, Puzhukkolli* • Telugu: *Nagamalle* • Kannada: *Nagamallige, Doddapatike* • Bengali: *Juipana* • Konkani: *Dadmari* • Urdu: *Palakjuhi* • Sanskrit: *Yudhikaparni, Yoodhikaparni*

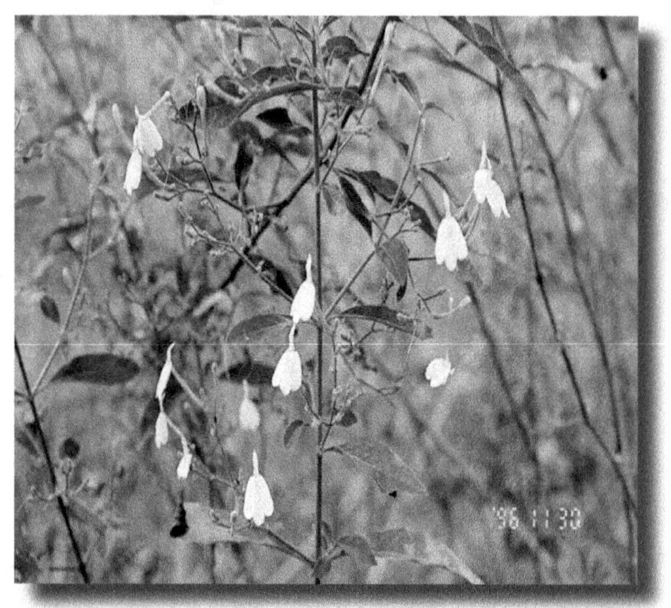

Description:
Native to India, this useful plant is a slender, erect, branched, somewhat hairy shrub 1-2 m in height. The leaves are oblong, 4-10 cm in length, and narrowed and pointed at both ends. The inflorescence is a spreading, leafy, hairy panicle with the flowers usually in clusters. The calyx is green, hairy, and about 5 mm long. The corolla-tube is greenish, slender, cylindric, and about 2 cm long. The flowers is 2-lipped; the upper lip is white, erect, oblong or lancelike, 2-toothed at the apex, and about 3 mm in both length and width; and the lower lip is broadly obovate, 1.1-1.3 cm in both measurements, 3-lobed, and white, with a few, minute, brownish dots near the base. The fruit (capsule) is club-shaped and contains four seeds.

Medicinal Uses:
In India the fresh roots and leaves, bruised and mixed with lime juice, are a useful remedy for ringworm and other skin affections. The seeds also are efficacious in ringworm. The root-bark is a remedy for dhobie's itch. In Sind, it is said to possess extraordinary aphrodisiacal powers, the roots boiled in milk being much employed by the Hindu practitioners. The roots are believed in some parts of India to be an antidote to the *bites of poisonous snakes.*

Karvy

Botanical Name:
Strobilanthes callosus

Family:
Acanthaceae **(Ruellia family)**

Synonyms:
Carvia callosa

Common Names:
Karvy • Hindi: *Maruadana* • Manipuri: *Khum* • Marathi: *Karvy*

Description:

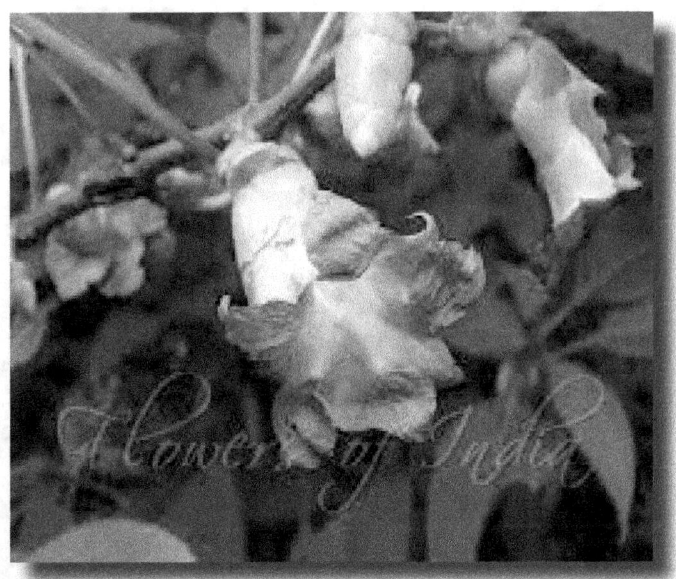

Karvy is a purplish-blue wild flower, which blooms once in every seven years. The plant was first discovered by Nees, a resident Britisher of Mumbai in the last century. The Karvy plant grows wild around Mumbai, Madhya Pradesh, Parts of Gujarat and in large areas of Konkan and North Kannara Ghats. It is a shrub growing 2-6 m tall. Oppositely arranged, elliptic-lancelike toothed leaves are 10-20 cm long. Each year the plant comes alive with the advent of Monsoon,and once the rains are over, what is left behind is dry and dead-looking stems.This pattern repeats itself for seven years. In the seventh year, the plant explodes into mass flowering. The Karvy plant has many uses as well. The leaves and the stems are also used for thatched roofs after the season is over.

Medicinal Uses:
The Karvy leaves are crushed and the juice is believed to be a sure cure for *stomach ailments*.

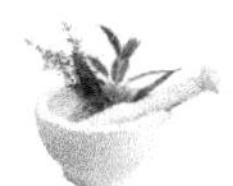

Singkrang

Botanical Name:

Saurauia roxburghii

Family:

Actinidiaceae **(Chinese Gooseberry family)**

Common Names:

Singkrang • Manipuri: *Singkrang* • Mizo: *Terpui* • Bengali: *Bon posola*

Description:

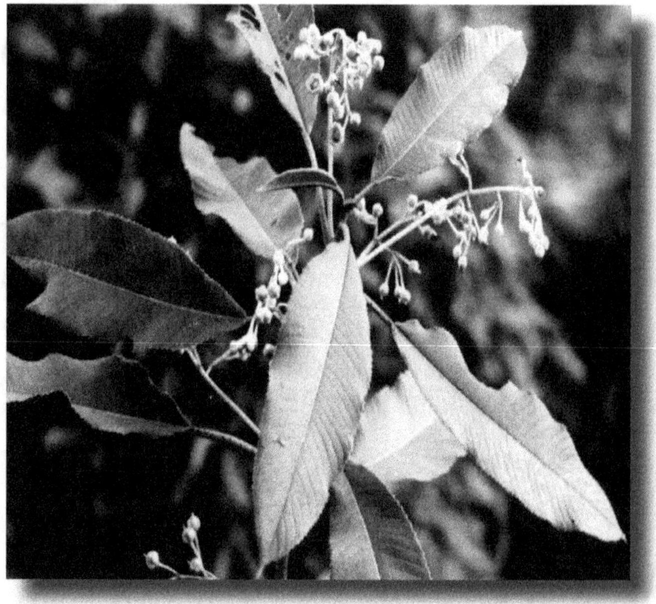

Singkrang is an evergreen tree, commonly found in North-east India - Manipur, Mizoram, Assam, etc. The tree is distinguished by its large elliptic leaves which are conspicuously rusty-haired beneath. Flowers arise in lax clusters of pink flowers. Flowers are very numerous, and the buds looks like *pink balls.* Sepals are whitish, unlike a similar, better known species Saurauia *napaulensis,* where the sepals are dark pink. Petals are five in number, pink, strongly overlapping, giving a cup shape to the open flower. Flowers generally hang looking down. Flowering: May-August.

Medicinal Uses:

A gummy or gelatinous substance produced by the leaves is used for preparing *hair pomade.*

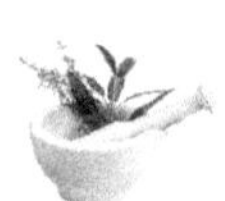

Sage Leaved Alangium

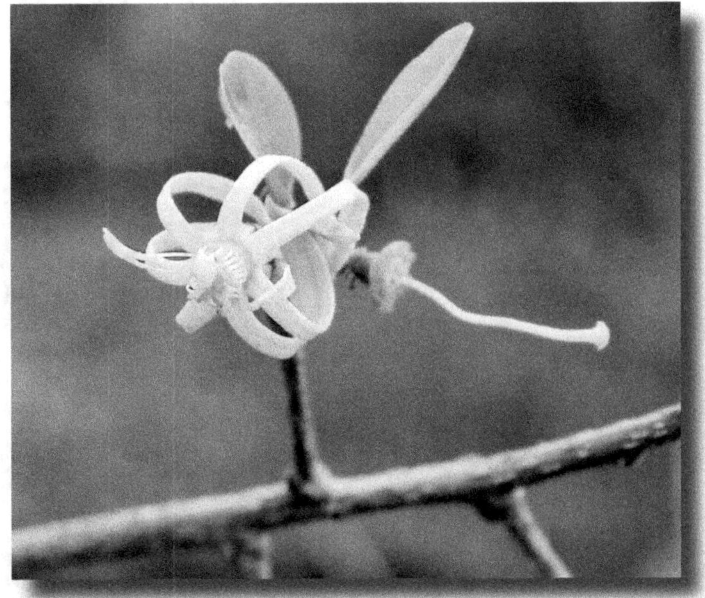

Botanical Name:

Alangium salviifolium

Family:

Alangiaceae (**Alangium family**)

Common Names:

Sage Leaved Alangium • Hindi: *Ankol* • Urdu: *Ankula* • Malayalam: *Arinjl* • Telugu: *Urgu* • Kannada: *Ankolamara* • Sanskrit: *Ankolah* • Tamil: *Alandi*

Description:

Sage Leaved Alangium is a tall thorny tree native to India. It grows to a height of about 3 to 10 metres. The bark is ash coloured, rough and faintly fissured. The leaves are elliptic oblong, elliptic lanceolate or oblong lanceolate. The flowers are greenish white, fascilcled, axillary or on old wood. The berries are ovoid, ellipsoid or nearly globose-glabrous, smooth and violet to purple. The flowering season is February to June.

Medicinal Uses:

In Ayurveda, the roots and the fruits are used for the treatment of *rheumatism* and *haemorrhoid*. Externally, it is used for the treatment of *bites of rabbits, rats* and *dogs*.

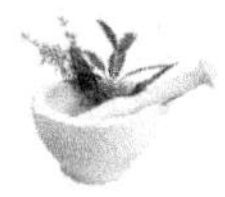

Chives

Botanical Name:
Allium schoenoprasum

Family:
Alliaceae (Onion family)

Common Names:
Chives • Hindi: *Chhoti pyaz* • Manipuri: *Tilhou macha*

Description:
Chives are a species of flowering plant in the onion family Alliaceae, native to Europe and Asia. They are referred to only in the plural, because they grow in clumps rather than alone. Chives are hardy, draught tolerant, perennials, eight

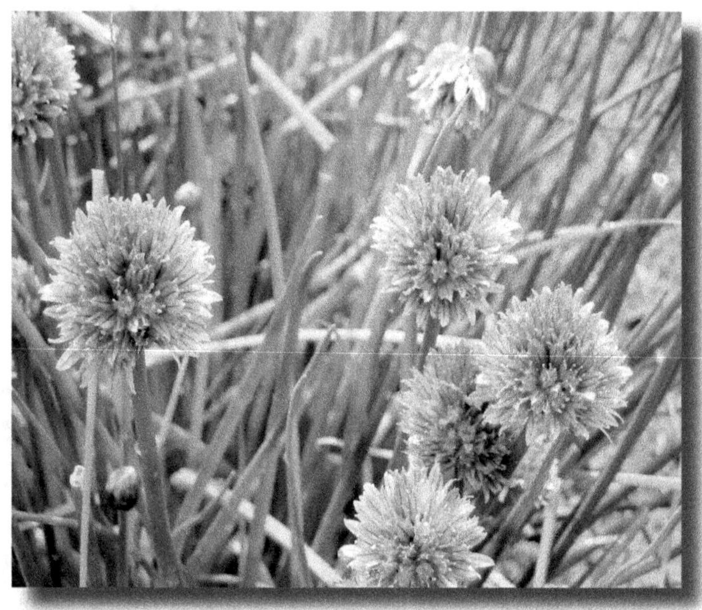

to twenty inches tall, that grow in clumps from underground bulbs. The leaves are round and hollow, similar to onions, but smaller in diameter. In June or July, chives produce large round flower heads consisting of purple to pink flowers. The flowers, which bloom for two months in midsummer, form round deep purple or pink globes that make an attractive garnish. Chives are grown for their leaves, which are used as a vegetable or a herb; they have a somewhat milder flavour than onions, green onions or garlics. Among the latter three Allium plants, the Chives resemble most the odour of green onions.

Medicinal Uses:
The ancient Chinese are the first documented to be using Chives, as long ago as 3000 years B.C. The Romans believed chives could relieve the *pain from sunburn* or a *sore throat*. They believed that eating chives would *increase blood pressure* and *acted as a diuretic.*

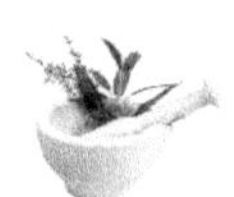

Himalayan Onion

Botanical Name:
Allium wallichii

Family:
Alliaceae (Onion family)

Common Names:
Himalayan Onion, Jimbur

Description:
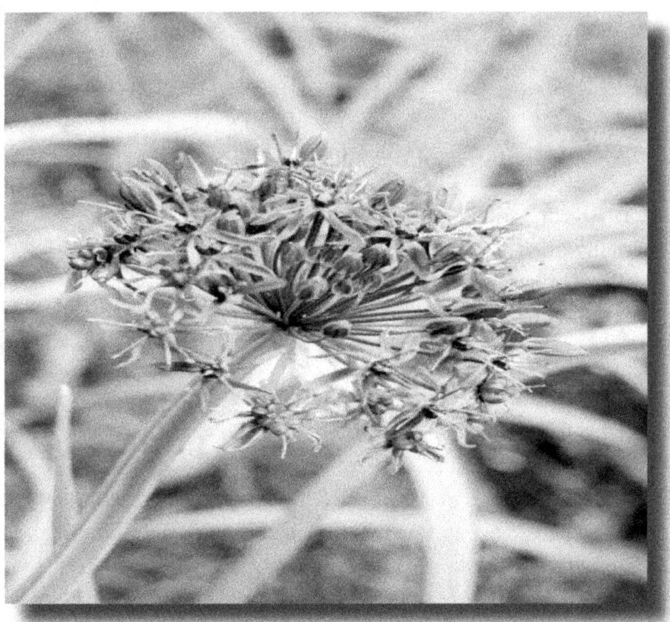

The Himalayan Onion is a *deciduous bulb* that grows to 1.0 meters high by 0.5 metres wide. It grows in Himalyan foothills between 2300-6600 m. It sports hemispheric umbels of purple flowers. In Nepal, Himalaya onion is often used for cooking, especially for flavouring (dal) boiled legumes. Rather uniquely, jimbu leaves are usually employed in the dried state and fried in butter fat to develop their flavour.

Medicinal Uses:
The bulbs, boiled then fried in ghee, are eaten in the treatment of *cholera* and *dysentery*. The raw bulb is chewed to treat *coughs* and *colds*. It is said that eating the bulbs can ease the symptoms of altitude sickness. Members of this genus are in general very healthy additions to the diet. They contain sulphur compounds (which give them their onion flavour) and when added to the diet on a regular basis they help *reduce blood cholesterol levels*, act as *a tonic to the digestive system* and also *tonify the circulatory system*.

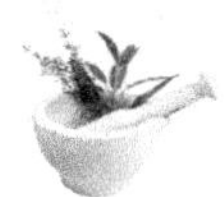

Prickly Chaff Flower

Botanical Name:
Achyranthes aspera

Family:
Amaranthaceae (**Amaranth family**)

Common Names:
Prickly Chaff Flower, Chaff-flower, Crocus stuff, Crokars staff, Devil's horsewhip • Hindi: *Chirchita, Latjira* • Manipuri: *Khujumpere* • Sanskrit: *Apamarga*

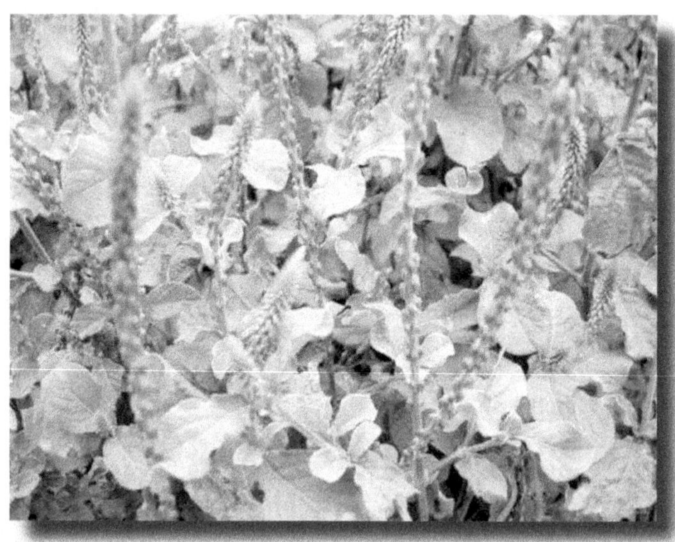

Description:
Prickly Chaff-flower is an erect or prostrate, annual or perennial herb, often with a woody base, which grows as wasteland herb every where. Since times immemorial, it is in use as folk medicine. It holds a reputed position as medicinal herb in different systems of medicine in India. Stems 0.4–2 m, pilose or puberulent. Leaf blades elliptic, ovate, or broadly ovate to orbiculate, obovate-orbiculate, or broadly rhombate, 1-20 × 2-6 cm, adpressed-pubescent abaxially and adaxially. Inflorescences to 30 cm; bracts membranous; bracteoles long-aristate, spinose; wings attached at sides and base. Flowers: tepals 4 or 5, length 3-7 mm; pseudostaminodes with margins fimbriate at apex, often with dorsal scale. According to the Black Yajurveda, Indra, having killed Vritra and other demons was overcome by Namuchi and made peace with him, promising never to kill him with any solid or liquid, neither by day or by night. But Indra collected some foam, which is neither solid nor liquid, and killed Namuchi in the morning between night and daybreak. From the head of the demon sprung the herb Apamarga, with the assistance of which Indra was able to kill all demons. Hence, this plant has the reputation of being a powerful talisman, and is now popularly supposed to act as a safeguard against *scorpions and snakes by paralysing them.*

Medicinal Uses:

The different parts of the plant are ingredients in many native prescriptions in combination with more active remedies. In Western India, the juice is applied to *relieve toothaches.* The ashes with honey are given to relieve cough; the root in dosed of *one tola* is given at bedtime for night blindness, and rubbed into a paste with water, it is used as an *anjan* (eye salve) in opacities of the cornea. The seeds are often used as a famine food in India, especially in the Rajputana, where the plant is called *Bharotha* (grass).

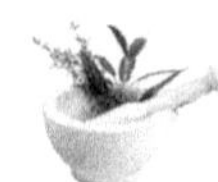

Two-toothed Chaff Flower

Botanical Name:
Achyranthes bidentata

Family:
Amaranthaceae (**Amaranth family**)

Common Names:
Two-toothed Chaff Flower, Ox knee, Pig's knee • Tamil: *Sigappu Nayurivi* • Sanskrit: *Apamarga* • Nepali: *Datiun, Rato apamarga*

Description:
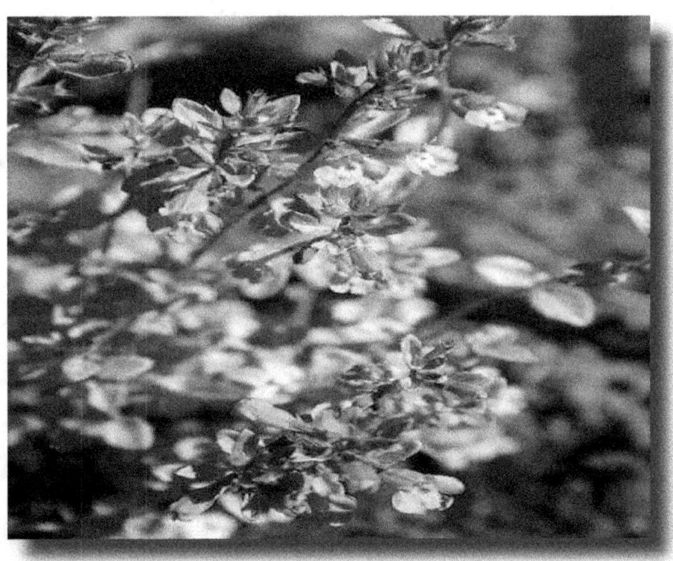

Two-toothed Chaff Flower is an erect, perennial herb, 0.7-1.2 m tall, distributed in hilly districts of India, Java, China and Japan. Stem green or tinged purple, with opposite branches. Leaf stalk 0.5-3 cm, hairy; leaf blade elliptic or elliptic-lanceolate, rarely oblanceolate, 4.5-12 × 2-7.5 cm. Flower spikes terminal or axillary, 3-5 cm; rachis 1-2 cm, white hairy. Flowers dense, 5 mm. Tepals shiny, lanceolate, 3-5 mm, with a midvein, apex acute. Stamens 2-2.5 mm; pseudostaminodes slightly serrulate, apex rounded. Utricles yellowish brown, shiny, oblong, 2-2.5 mm, smooth. Seeds light brown, oblong, 1 mm. Seed are cooked and eaten. A good substitute for cereal grains in bread-making, they have often been used for this purpose during famine. Flowering: July-September. *Leaves* are used as a *vegetable* in the same manner as *spinach*.

Medicinal Uses:
It is a Traditional Chinese Herb used to *nourish the kidney and liver, drain 'dampness'* and *promote circulation*. It is prescribed for *difficult urination, painful urethritis and suppressed menstruation*. Commonly used to treat traumatic injuries, stiffness and pain of the lower back and loins and for weakness in the legs and feet. *Do not use during pregnancy.*

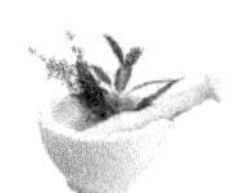

Mountain Knot Grass

Botanical Name:

Aerva lanata

Family:

Amaranthaceae (**Amaranth family**)

Synonyms:

Aerva elegans, Illecebrum lanatum, Achyranthes lanata

Common Names:

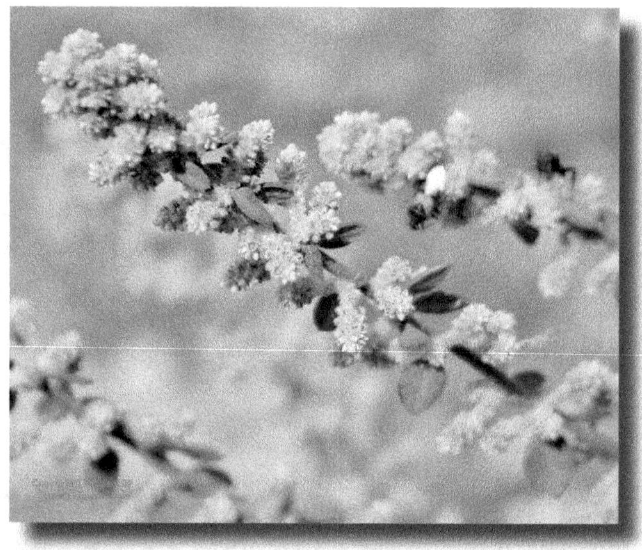

Mountain Knot Grass • Hindi: *Chhaya, Gorakhbuti, Gorakhganja, Kapurijadi, Khali, Khari* • Marathi: *Kapurmadhuri* • Tamil: *Cirupulai, Ulinai* • Malayalam: *Cherula* • Telugu: *Pindidonda* • Kannada: *Bili himdi soppu* • Bengali: *Chaya* • Rajasthani: *Bhui* • Konkani: *Tamdlo* • Punjabi: *Bui-kaltan* • Sanskrit: *Ashmahabhedah, Bhadra, Gorakshaganja, Pashanabheda, Shatakabhedi*

Description:

Mountain Knot Grass is a perennial herb, occasionally woody below, prostrate to erect, 0.3-2 m, branched from the base and often also from above. Stem and branches are densely woolly with whitish or yellowish, shaggy hairs. Alternately arrange leaves are nearly circular to lanceshaped-elliptic, wedge-shaped at the base, rounded to sharp at the tip. Leaves are usually densely woolly on the lower surface and more thinly so above. Leaves on the main stem are 1-5 cm long, 0.5-3.5 cm wide, those of the branches and upper part of the stem are smaller. Leaf stalks are up to 2 cm. Flower spikes are stalkless, solitary or usually in clusters in leaf axils, 0.4-1.5 cm long, 3-4 mm wide, divergent, cylindrical, silky white to creamy, forming a long inflorescence leafy to the ultimate spikes.

Medicinal Uses:

This herb is described as one of the best known remedies for *bladder and kidney stones*. Ayurvedic practitioners recommend a *decoction of the plant to be taken internally for a few days to dissolve the stone and to clear the urinary path.*

Sessile Joyweed

Botanical Name:
Alternanthera sessilis

Family:
Amaranthaceae (**Amaranth family**)

Common Names:
Sessile Joyweed, Dwarf copperleaf, Joyweed • Hindi: *Garundi, Guroo* • Manipuri: *Phakchet* • Marathi: *Kanchari* • Tamil: *Ponnanganni* • Malayalam: *Ponnankannikkira* • Telugu: *Ponnagantikura* • Kannada: *Honagonne* • Oriya: *Madaranga* • Konkani: *Koypa* • Sanskrit: *Matsyaksi*

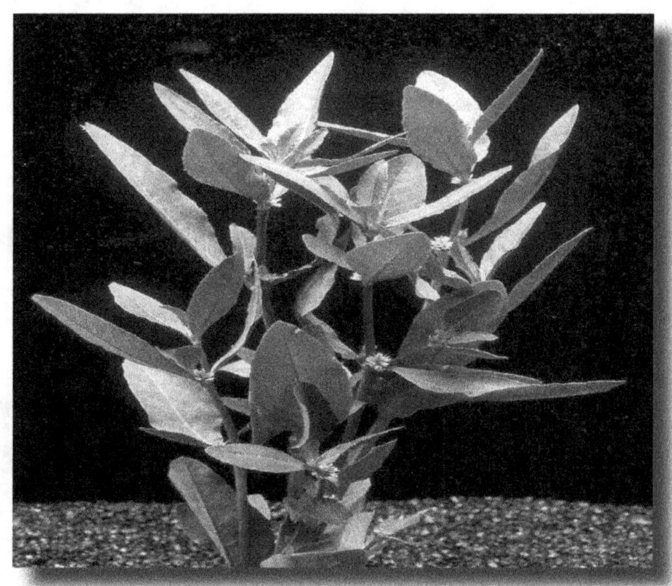

Description:
Sessile Joyweed is a perennial herb, often found in and near ponds, canals and reservoirs. It prefers places with constant or periodically high humidity and so may be found in swamps, shallow ditches, and fallow rice fields. A much branched prostrate herb, branches often purplish, frequently rooting at the lower nodes; leaves simple, opposite, somewhat fleshy, lanceolate, oblanceolate or linear-oblong, obtuse or subacute, sometimes obscurely denticulate, glabrous, shortly petiolate; flowers small, white, in axillary clusters; fruits compressed obcordate utricles, seeds suborbicular.

Medicinal Uses:
The stems and leaves of this plant are useful in *eye trouble*. Decoction is taken with little salt drunk to check *vomiting of blood*. The shoot with other ingredients are used to *restore virility*. The poultice is used for *boils*.

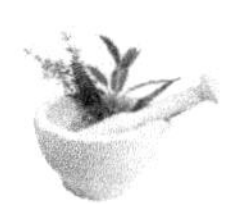

Milk and Wine Lily

Botanical Name:
Crinum latifolium

Family:
Amaryllidaceae (**Nargis family**)

Synonyms:
Crinum zeylanicum

Common Names:
Milk and Wine Lily, Ceylon swamplily, Pink striped trumpet lily • Hindi: Sudarshan • Marathi: Gandani-kanda, Gadambhikanda, Golkamdo • Tamil: Vishamungil • Kannada: Vish mungli • Bengali: Sukhdarshan • Konkani: Golkando • Sanskrit: Madhuparnika, Vrishakarni

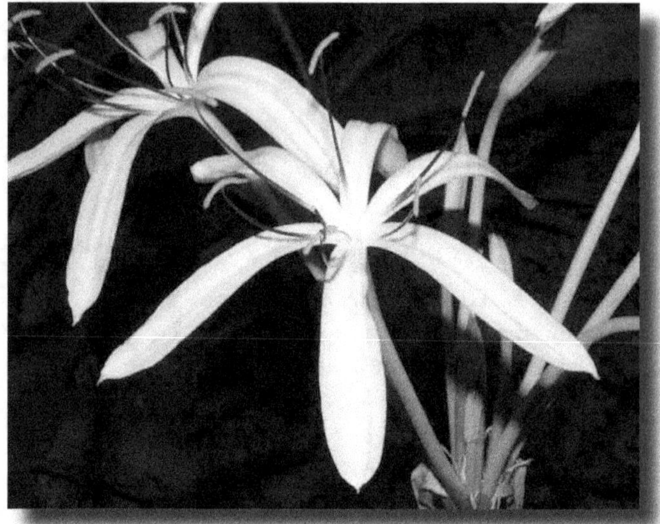

Description:
This old fashioned crinum lily is a low maintence plant that produces lovely, large, striped, lily-like flowers. The stripes are alternately wine pink and white. The flowers also have a wonderful faintly sweet fragrance. The tall bloom stalk stands about 18-24 inches above the abundant foilage and hold 5+ blooms at a time! These will produce several flower stalks during the warmer months with the majority of blooms coming in the spring and fall. These lilies will multiply by producing bulbs underground as well as from the seeds that form after the blooms. You'll have a lovely large group of these in no time. Milk and Wine Lily are native to India. Flowering: June-August.

Medicinal Uses:
Bulbs are *extremely acrid.* When roasted, they are used as a *rubefacient in rheumatism.* Crushed and toasted bulb is applied to *piles* and *abscesses* to cause suppuration. The juice of the leaf is used in *earaches.*

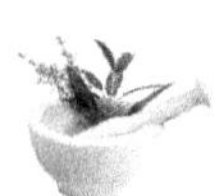

Marking Nut

Botanical Name:

Semecarpus anacardium

Family:

Anacardiaceae (**Cashew family**)

Synonyms:

Anacardium orientale

Common Names:

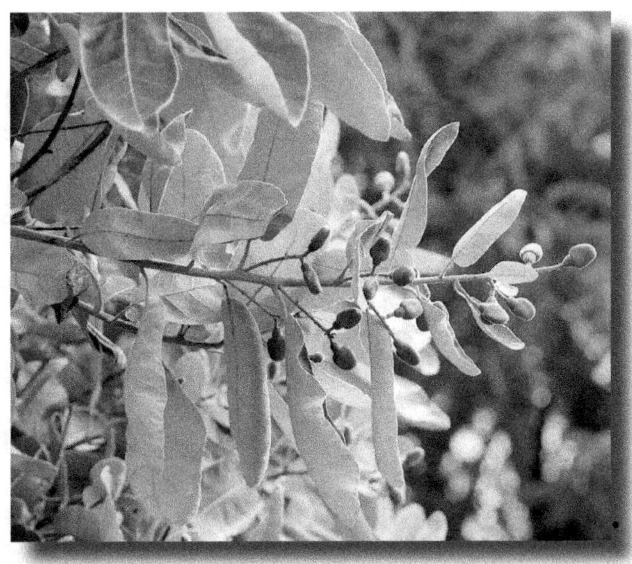

Marking Nut, Dhobi nut tree, Indian marking nut tree, Malacca bean, Marany nut, Marsh nut, Oriental cashew nut, Varnish tree • Hindi: *Bhilawan, Billar* • Marathi: *Bhallataka, Bhillava, Bibba* • Tamil: *Cen-kottai, Compalam, Kalakam, Kavaka, Kitta-k-kani-k-kottai* • Malayalam: *Alakuceer, Ceenkkuru, Theenkotta* • Telugu: *Bhallatamu, Jidimamidichettu* • Kannada: *Geru, Gerannina mara* • Bengali: *Bhallata, Bhallataka* • Oriya: *Bhollataki, Bonebhalia* • Konkani: *Amberi, Bibba* • Urdu: *Baladur, Bhilavan, Billar* • Assamese: *Bhala* • Gujarati: *Bhilamo, Bhilamu* • Sanskrit: *Ahvala, Arshastah, Arudhkh, Bhallatakah, Vahnih, Vishasya* • Nepali: *Bhalaayo*

Description:

Marking Nut is a moderate-sized deciduous tree with large stiff leaves. Leaves are 7-24 inches long, 2-12 inches wide, obovate-oblong, rounded a t the tip. Leaf base is rounded, heart-shaped or narrowed into the stalk, leathery in texture. Flowers is small, borne in panicles shorter than the leaves. Fruit is a drupe 1 inch long, ovoid or oblong, smooth and shining, black when ripe, seated on a fleshy cup. The stem yields, by tapping, an acrid, viscid juice from which a varnish is prepared. The nut yields a powerful and bitter substance used everywhere in India as a substitute for marking ink for clothes by washermen, hence it is frequently called Dhobi Nut. It gives a black colour to cotton fabrics, but before application it must be mixed with limewater as a fixator. The fruits are also used as a *dye*. They are also largely employed in *Indian medicine*. The *fleshy cups* on which the nuts rest and the *kernels of the nuts* are eaten.

Medicinal Uses:

The fruit is useful in *leucoderma, scaly skin, allergic, dermatitis, poisonous bites, leprosy, cough, asthma,* and *dyspepsia*. It is extremely beneficial in diseases like *piles, colitis, diarrhoea, dyspepsia, ascites, tumours* and *worms*. The topical application of its oil on *swollen joints* and *traumatic wounds* effectively *controls the pain*.

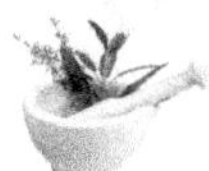

Sugar Apple

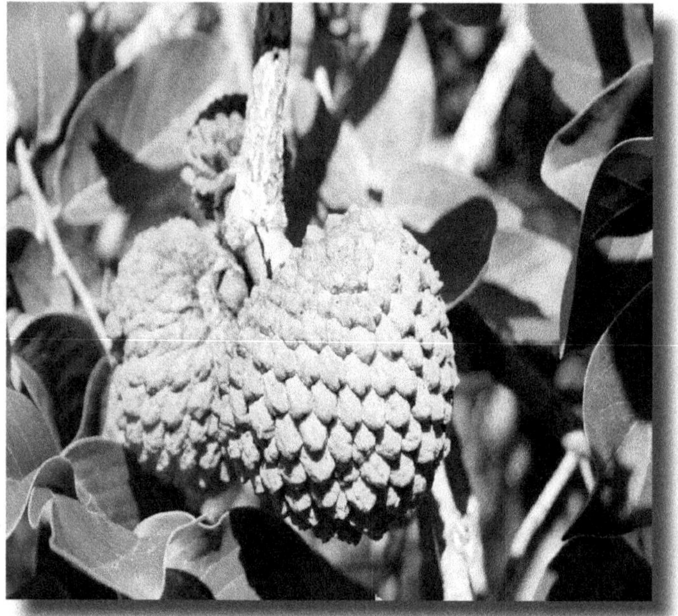

Botanical Name:

Annona squamosa

Family:

Annonaceae (Sugar apple family)

Common Names:

Sugar Apple, Custard apple • Hindi: Sharifa , Sitaphal • Manipuri: Sitaphal • Assamese: Katal • Tamil: Sitapalam

Description:

A small tropical tree, indigenous to the Amazon rainforest, growing up to 20' tall. The leaves are thin, oblong while the flowers are greenish - yellow. Flowers are oblong, 1 to 1 1/2 in long, never fully open, with 1 in long, drooping stalks, and 3 fleshy outer petals, yellow-green on the outside and pale-yellow inside with a purple or dark-red spot at the base. The avoid or conical fruit, with a purple knobby skin, is very sweet and is eaten fresh or can be used for shakes. The fruit is juicy and creamy - white; it may contain up to 40 black seeds. These seeds are poisonous. From delicious fruits of Sitaphal, jelly, jam, conserves, sharbets, syrup, tart and fermented drinks are prepared. The peelings and pulps contain oil that is useful in flavouring.

Medicinal Uses:

The bark and leaves contain annonaine, an alkaloid. In tropical America, a decoction of the leaves is used as a cold remedy and to clarify urine. A bark decoction is used to stop diarrhea, while the root is used in the treatment of dysentery.

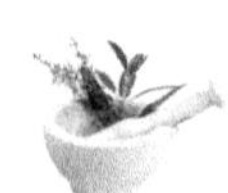

Himalayan Thorowax

Botanical Name:
Bupleurum candollei

Family:
Apiaceae (**Carrot family**)

Common Names:
Himalayan Thorowax, Bupleurum, Hare's Ear, Thorowax Root

Description:
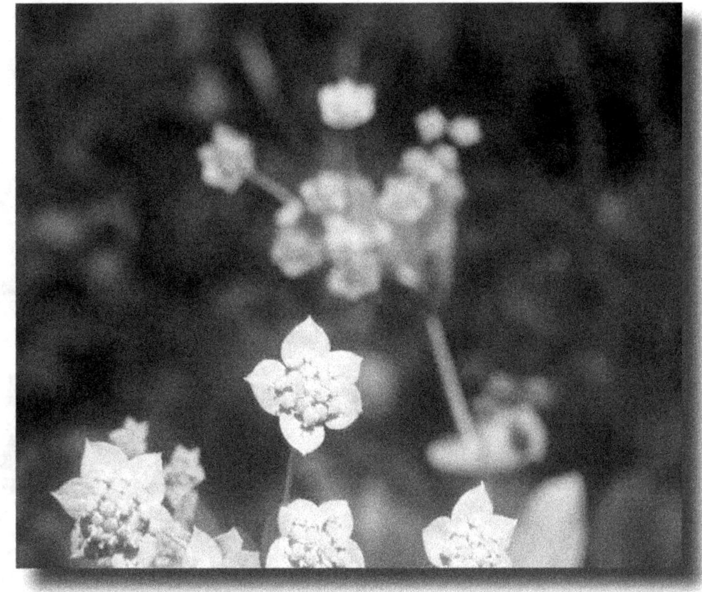

The Himalayan Thorowax is a medicinal plant whose Chinese cousin is popular in Chinese medicine. It is an erect perennial herb which grow upto 1 m high. Oblong-ovate stem leaves are almost without stalk, and have an smooth margin. Tiny flowers appear in compound umbels 2.5–4 cm across, typical of the carrot family. The flowers themselves are very small, and appear in a bunch of 10-15 in secondary umbels 8–12 mm across, enclosed in unequal bracts which looks like leaves. The flowers petals are either pale yellow or dark purple. Himalayan Thorowax are found in mixed forests on shady slopes, open forests, mountain slopes, grassy places, at altitudes 2400–4000 m. This genus is very confusing and the species are highly variable.

Medicinal Uses:
The roots of several species of Bupleurum are famous for their use as traditional Chinese medicine, 'chai hu' for treatment of *coughs, fevers* and *influenza*. Almost all of the species are recorded in the literature as regional substitutes for 'chai hu' or for other local medicinal purposes. However, caution should be applied, as very few species are toxic (e.g., B. longiradiatum) and can result in 'toxic strike' if misused as such substitutes.

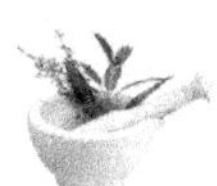

Indian Pennywort

Botanical Name:
Centella asiatica

Family:
Apiaceae (**Carrot family**)

Common Names:
Indian Pennywort, Coinwort, Asiatic coinwort, American coinwort, spadeleaf • Hindi: *Brahma manduki* • Malayalam: *Kodangal* • Kannada: *Vondelaga* • Tamil: *Vallarai* • Assamese: *Bor-mani-muni* • Manipuri: *Peruk* • Telugu: *Saraswataku* • Bengali: *Bora thulkari* • Marathi: *Karinga*

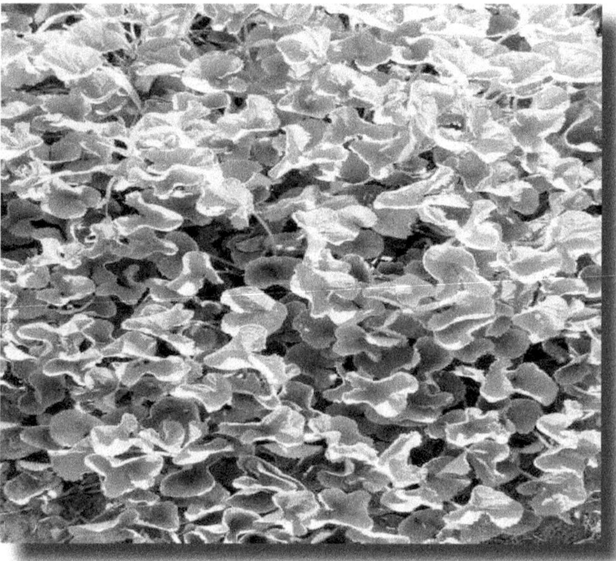

Description:
Indian Pennywort is a small creeping herb with shovel shaped leaves emerging alternately in clusters at the stem nodes. The runners lie along the ground and the inch long leaves with their scalloped edges rise above on long reddish petioles. The insignificant greenish- to pinkish-white flowers are borne in dense umbels (clusters in which all the flower stalks arise from the same point) on separate stems in the summer. The seeds are pumpkin-shaped nutlets 0.1-0.2 in long. In India it is revered as a medicinal herb, and particularly in Manipur the full plant is eaten as food like a leafy vegetable. Indian Pennywort appears to have originated in the wetlands of Asia. China, India and Malaya were probably within its original range.

Medicinal Uses:
The Indian Pennywort is revered as one of the greatest *multi-purpose miracle herbs of Oriental medicine*. It has been in use for thousands of years and has been employed to treat *practically every ailment* known to man at one time or place or another. The leaf and root extract has been used in *Ayurvedic medicine* for a long time but has become very popular in the past couple of years for both internal use as well as topical application - although the cosmetic application is relatively new. In Ayurvedic practice, it also has a valuable and sought-after *Vayasthapana effect* - helping to *retard the aging process*.

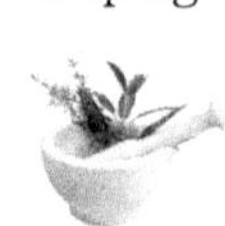

Himalayan Hogweed

Botanical Name:
Heracleum lallii

Family:
Apiaceae (**Carrot family**)

Common Names:
Himalayan Hogweed, Hogweed

Description:
This *beautiful flower* from the carrot family adorns the *Valley of Flowers* in uttarakhand (India) with its typical *carrot like white flowers appearing in dense umbels.*

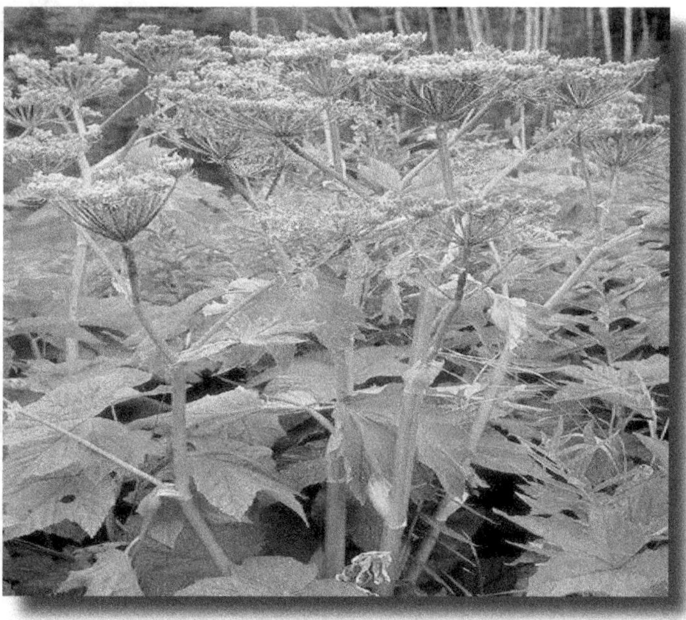

Medicinal Uses:
The root is used in *Tibetan medicine,* where it is considered to have a bitter and acrid taste with a neutral potency. *Analgesic, anthelmintic* and *anti-inflammatory,* it is used in the treatment of *contagious diseases, swelling/pain* in *the joints* and *arthritis.* It is also used in the treatment of *all types of pains, toothaches* and for the *inability* to *defecate.*

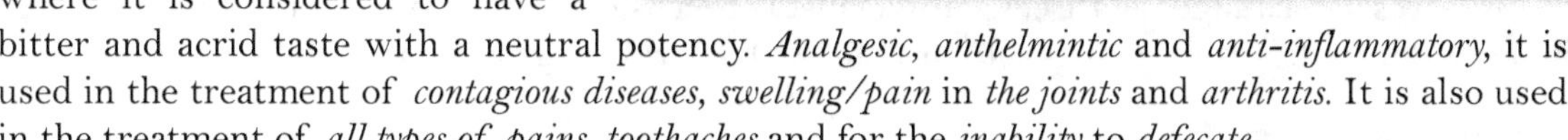

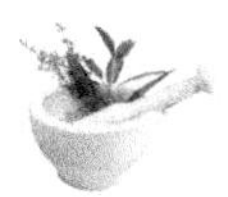

Nepal Hogweed

Botanical Name:
Heracleum nepalense

Family:
Apiaceae (**Carrot family**)

Common Names:
Nepal *Hogweed* • Nepali: *Budho Aushaadhi*

Description:
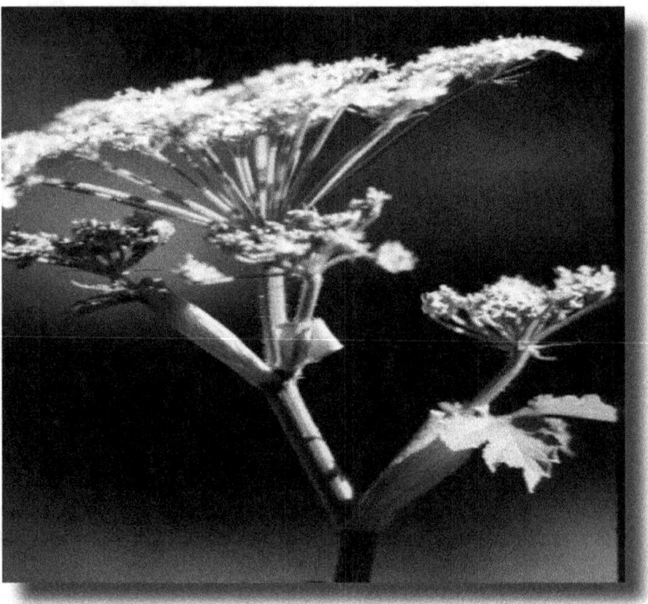

Nepal Hogweed is a small shrub which grows from Himachal Pradesh to Bhutan. It is somewhat similar to the Himalayan Hogweed. The stems can grow to 60-160 cm tall. Lower leaves are pinnate with toothed, deeply lobed, or pinnately-cut large leaflets. The upper leaves are arranged in threes, with lelaflets often 3-lobed. Flowers are small, white, borne in upright umbels. Fruits are obovate to 1 cm, with lateral wings and weak ribs.

Medicinal Uses:
Nepal Hogweed is used in *veterinary medicine*. It exhibits stimulant property and increases the rate of respiration and blood pressure in goats. The root of the plant is used as a *digestive, an aphrodisiac, a carminative and an antidiarrhoeal in folk medicine.*

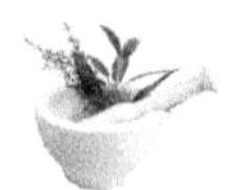

Wild Carrot

Botanical Name:
Peucedanum grande

Family:
Apiaceae (**Carrot family**)

Common Names:
Wild Carrot • Hindi: *Daku, Duku* • Marathi: *Baphali* • Urdu: *Daku* • Sanskrit: *Baspika, Ela*

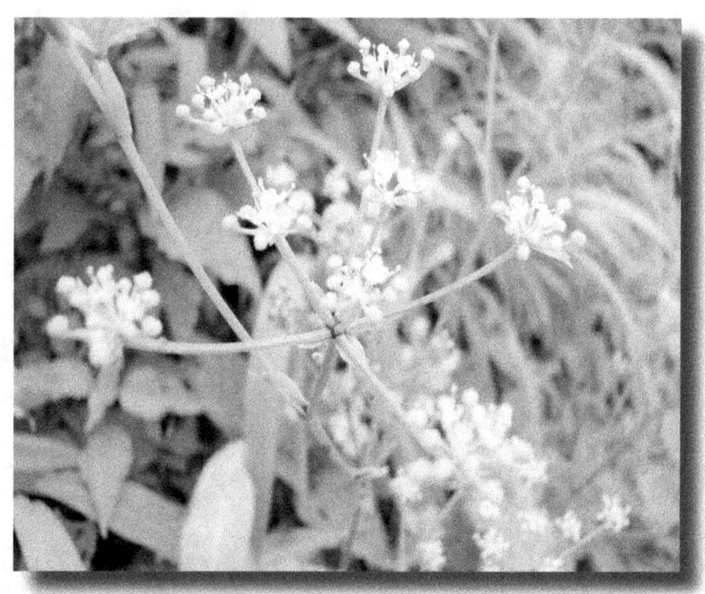

Description:
Wild Carrot is a herb from the carrot family. it is an erect herb 3-4 ft in height, with yellow flowers arranged in a compound umbel. It flowers during the later half of the monsoons. The fruit is used in curries as a flavouring agent. Wild Carrot is found in the Western Ghats.

Medicinal Uses:
The infusion of the fruit is used in doses of half to 1 ounce like that of fennel seeds, as carminative, diuretic and stimulant in *flatulency, gastric* and *intestinal disorders,* etc.

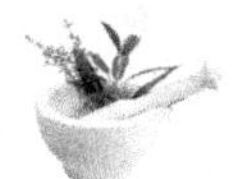

Batino

Botanical Name:

Alstonia macrophylla

Family:

Apocynaceae (**Oleander family**)

Common Names:

Batino, Devil-tree, Hard alstonia • Marathi: *Mothi Saatveen* • Kannada: *Janthaala mara*

Description:

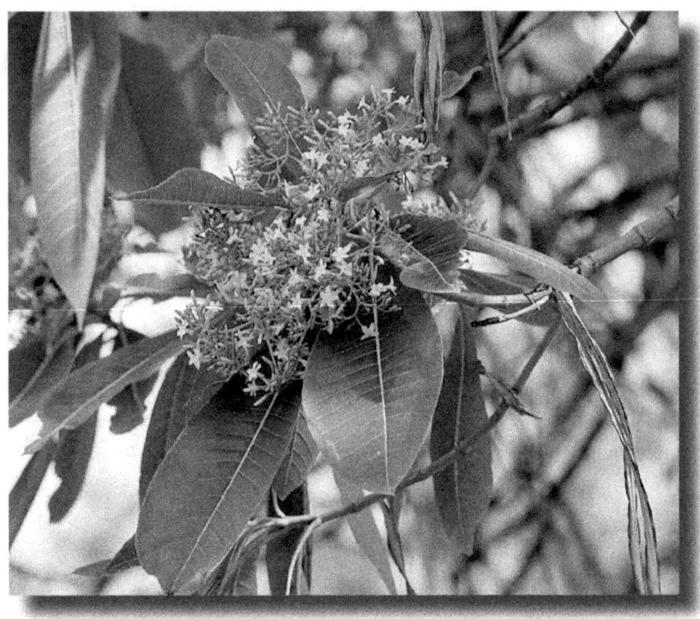

Batino is common in forests and thickets at low and medium altitudes in many parts of South-East Asia. It was first introduced in *India and Sri Lanka*. It is a *medium-sized evergreen tree*. The leaves are in whorls of three, oblong-obovate, 10-30 cm long, 5-7 cm wide, pointed at both ends, and short-stalked.

The flowers are small, yellowish-white, and borne on short cymes at the end of branches. The sepal cup is small. The flowers consist of a 1–1.5 cm long tube, opening into 5 pure-white petals. The fruit is a double follicle, pendant, very long, and slender, being 20-40 cm long. The seeds are small and very flat, with deep-brown, especially along the edges.

Medicinal Uses:

In Philippines, the bark, in the form of powder, decoction, infusion, tincture, or wine preparation, is used as a febrifuge, a tonic, an antiperiodic and antidysenteric.

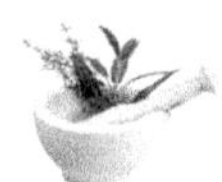

Sea Mango

Botanical Name:
Cerbera manghas

Family:
Apocynaceae (**Oleander family**)

Synonyms:
Cerbera venenifera, Tanghinia venenifera

Common Names:
Sea Mango, Madagascar ordeal bean, Odollam tree, Pink-eyed cerbera, Dog-bane • Marathi: *Sukanu* • Tamil: *Kodalma, Kattarali, Kottuma, Caat aralie* Malayalam: *Utalam, Chattankaya* • Kannada: *Chande, Monde*

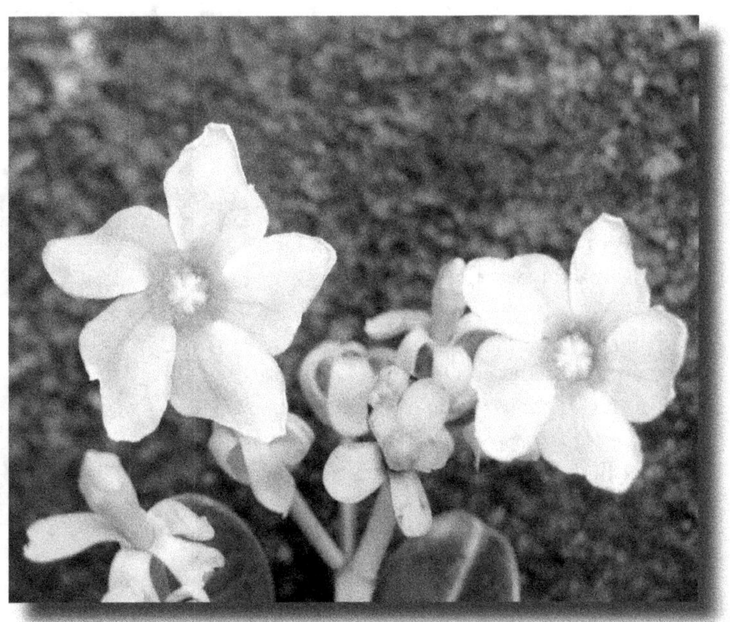

Description:
Sea Mango is a small evergreen coastal tree growing up 12 m tall. The shiny dark-green leaves are alternate ovoid in shape. The flowers are fragrant, possessing a white tubular five lobed corolla about 3 to 5 cm in diameter, with a pink to red throat. They have five stamens and the ovary is positioned above the other flower parts. The fruits are egg-shaped, 5-10 cm long, and turn bright red at maturity. Sea Mango is native to Madagascar, South-East Asia, and many Pacific islands. Flowering: April-August.

Medicinal Uses:
The seed oil in plasters applied to the skin is effective for scabies and prurigo, and when applied to the hair kills *head-lice*. The glycosides extracted from the seeds are active on *heart failure*. The trunk bark or the leaves are occasionally used as a *purgative*, but strict precautions must be taken because of their *high toxicity*.

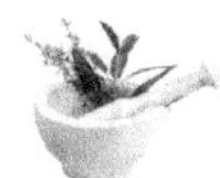

Indrajao

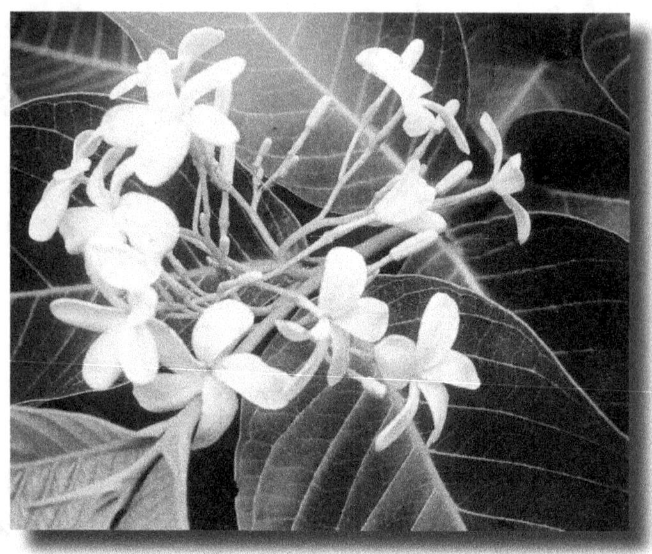

Botanical Name:

Holarrhena pubescens

Family:

Apocynaceae (**Oleander family**)

Synonyms:

Holarrhena antidysenterica

Common Names:

Indrajao • Assamese: Dhulkari, Dudkhuri • Bengali: *Kurchi, Kutaja* • Gujarati: *Kadavo indrajav* • Hindi: *Karva indrajau, Kutaja* • Kannada: *Koodsaloo, Korchie* • Kashmiri: *Andusurun* • Konkani: Kudo • Malayalam: Kutakappaala • Marathi: Indrajav, Kutaja, Pandhra kuda • Punjabi: Keor, *Kewar* • Oriya: *Kherwa, Korwa, Kurwa, Pitakorwa* • Sanskrit: *Indrayava, Kutaja, Sakraparyaaya, Sakraasana, vatsaka* • Tamil: *Kirimllikai, Kutaca-p-palai, Mlaimllikai* • Telugu: *Girimallika, Kodisepala, Kolamukku, Kondamalle, Kutajamu*

Description:

Indrajao is a deciduous shrub or a small tree, growing up to 3 ms high. Short stem has pale bark and several branches. Oppositely arranges, ovate, obtusely acuminate leaves are 10-20 cm long. Leaf stalks are very short. White flowers appear in corymb-like cymes, 5-15 cm across, at the end of branches. Flowers have five white petals 2-3 cm long which turn creamish yellow as they age. The flowers are beautiful with oblong petals which are rounded at the tip, and remind one of *frangipani*.

Medicinal Uses:

It is a medicinal plant in *Ayurveda*. One of its botanical synonyms *Holarrhena antidysenterica* says it all. It is one of the best drug for *Diarrhoea*. In *chronic diarrhoea* and to *check blood coming from stool*, it should be *given with Isobgol, caster oil* or *Indrayav*. According to *Ayurveda*, the bark is useful in treatment of *piles, skin diseases and biliousness*. The bark is used externally in case of skin troubles. Is is mostly mixed with cow urine and applied in affected parts. Is is used the treatment of urinary troubles and the bark is given with cows milk. The fresh juice of bark is considered good to check the diarrhoea. In bleeding piles, Decoction of *Kutaj bark* with *sunthi* checks *mucus and blood*. Application of this herb is useful in *Rh. Arthritis* and *Oestioarthritis*.

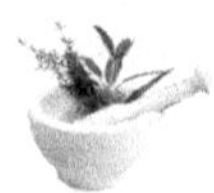

Shrub Vinca

Botanical Name:

Kopsia fruticosa

Family:

Apocynaceae **(Oleander family)**

Common Names:

Shrub Vinca, Pink Kopsia, Pink Gardenia • Bengali: *Dakur*

Description:

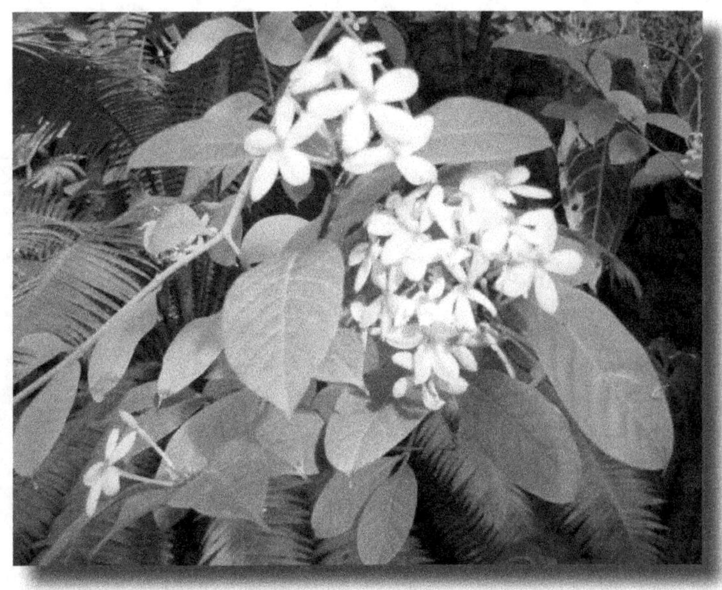

Shrub Vinca is a tall bush with simple leaves. It has an interesting resemblance to *Frangipani*. It is an evergreen shrub growing up to 4 m tall. The plant is hairless except for inflorescences. Leaf stalk is 1 cm. Leaf blade narrowly elliptic or narrowly oblong, 10-23 X 2.5-9 cm, tip sharp or blunt. Flowers occur in bunches of a few. Beautiful light pink flowers, which may also be almost white, have 5 petals that are oblong, 1.5-2.5 cm. The plant is distributed *in India, Indonesia, Malaysia, Philippines and Thailand*. It is cultivated as an ornamental plant as well as for its medicinal properties.

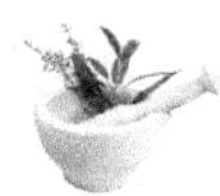

Sarpagandha

Botanical Name:
Rauvolfia serpentina

Family:
Apocynaceae (**Oleander family**)

Synonyms:
Rauwolfia serpentine

Common Names:
**Indian Snakeroot, Insanity herb •
Hindi:** *Sarpagandha*

Description:
Sarpagandha is a famous tranquilizer and antipsychotic herb of India for the treatment of *paranoia* and 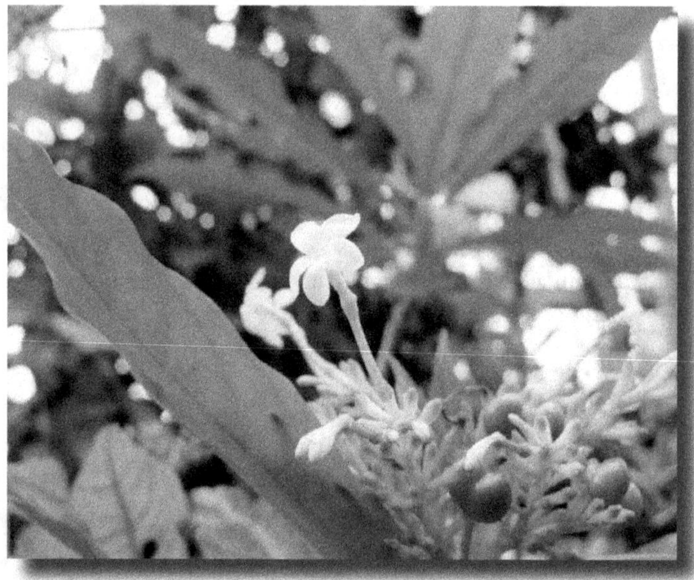 *schizophrenia*, as well as a substance that controls *hypertension*. Sarpagandha is an erect, evergreen shrub, merely 15 to 45 cm high. Its leaves are large, in whorls of three - dark green above and pale green below. The flowers are white, pinkish or red, occurring in whorls. Its fruit are tiny, oval, fleshy which turn a shiny purple-black when ripe. It is the roots of the plant that are mainly used for medicinal purposes.

Medicinal Uses:
Although this plant was well known in India, westerners paid no attention to it until an Indian physician wrote an article on rauvolfia in 1943. Because of the drug's noted sedative effects, it was used to treat over a million Indians in the 1940s for high blood pressure. After a U.S. physician named the plant, *Wilkins* demonstrated the positive effects of *Reserpine* (1952), the plant which made the front page news. This drug rapidly replaced *electric shock and lobotomy as treatments for certain types of mental illnesses.* Moreover, knowledge about the chemistry of this natural plant stimulated the synthesis of other similar alkaloids that are now used as major *tranquilizers.*

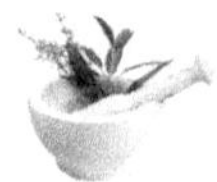

Wild Snake Root

Botanical Name:

Rauvolfia tetraphylla

Family:

Apocynaceae (**Oleander family**)

Synonyms:

Rauvolfia canescens, Rauvolfia heterophylla, Rauvolfia hirsute

Common Names:

Wild Snake Root, Devil Pepper, Be Still Tree, American serpentwood, Be still tree, Devil root, Milkbush • Hindi: *Barachandrika, Chandrabhaga* • Tamil: *Pampukaalaachchedi* • Malayalam: *Pampumkolli, Kattamalpori* • Telugu: *Papataku* • Kannada: *Dodda chandrike* • Bengali: *Bar chandrika, Gandhanakuli* • Oriya: *Patalagarudi* • Sanskrit: *Vanasarpagandha, Sarpanasini*

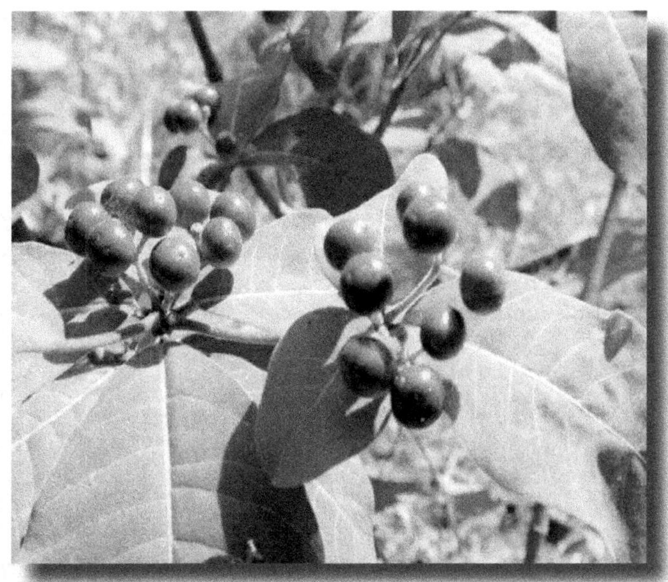

Description:

Native to tropical America, Wild Snake Root is a small tree or shrub that reaches a height of 6 ft. Leaves are whorled, medium to dark green in colour, and occur in groups of four unequally-sized leaves at each node. By late summer to early fall, the very small, white flowers appear. Flowers are 5 mm long, and the tube is 3.7 mm long. The fruits are bright red berries that turn black as they ripen, They look like large *pepper corns*.

Medicinal Uses:

The roots yield the drug *deserpidine*, which is an *antihypertensive* and *tranquilizer*.

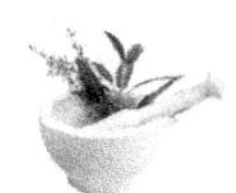

Nag Kuda

Botanical Name:

Tabernaemontana alternifolia

Family:

Apocynaceae (Oleander family)

Synonyms:

**Ervatamia heyneana,
Tabernaemontana heyneana**

Common Names:

Nag Kuda • Marathi: *Nag-kuda*
• Malayalam: *Churutu-pala,
Kampippala* • Sanskrit: *Kampillakah*

Description:

Nag Kuda is a small tree native to Western Ghats, growing up to 2-5 m tall. Oppositely arranged leaves

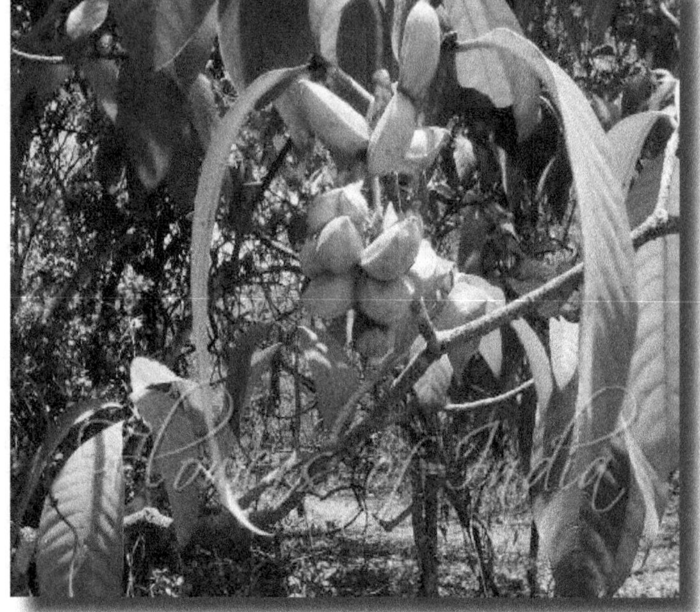

are elliptic-oblong, 23 cm long, 6.5 cm wide, prominently nerved. White flowers are borne in corymb-like cymes. Sepals are five in number, thick, fused at the base. Flowers have a narrow tube which flares into a flat flower. Five stamens do not protrude out. The fruit is quite interesting – it consists of two boat-shaped orange pods, up to 4 cm long, with recurved beaks.

Medicinal Uses:

This plant is used in *Ayurveda*.

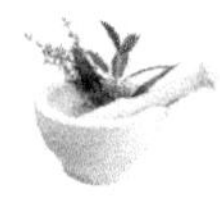

Sweet Indrajao

Botanical Name:
Wrightia tinctoria

Family:
Apocynaceae (**Oleander family**)

Common Names:
Sweet Indrajao, Pala indigo plant, Dyers's oleander • Hindi: *Kapar, Dudhi* • Tamil: *Paalai* • Marathi: *Kala kuda*

Description:
Sweet Indrajao is a small, deciduous tree with a light gray, scaly smooth bark. Native to India and Burma, Wrightia is Named after a Scottish

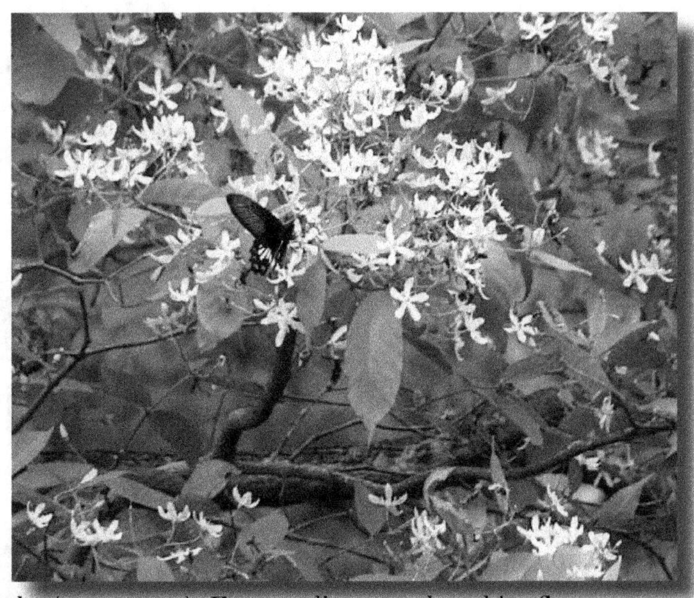

physician and botanist William Wright (1740-1827). From a distance, the white flowers may appear like *snow flakes* on a tree. The fruits as pendulous, long paired follicles joined at their tips. The hairy seeds are released as the fruit dehisces. The leaves of this tree yield a blue dye called *Pala Indigo*. Sweet Indrajao is called dhudi (Hindi) because of its preservative nature. Supposedly a few drops of its sap in milk *prevent curdling* and enhance its *shelf life*, without the need to *refrigerate*. The *wood* of Sweet Indrajao is extensively used for all classes of tannery. It is made into cups, plates, combs, pen holders, pencils and bed stead legs. It is commonly used for making *Chennapatna toys*.

Medicinal Uses:
The leaves are applied as a poultice for mumps and herpes and sometimes, they are also munched to relieve toothaches. In folk medicine, the dried and powdered roots of Wrightia along with Phyllanthus amarus (keezhanelli) and Vitex negundo (nochi) is mixed with milk and orally administered to women for improving fertility. *The bark and seeds are effective against psoriasis* and *non-specific dermatitis*. It has anti-inflammatory and anti-dandruff properties and hence, is used in *hair oil preparations*.

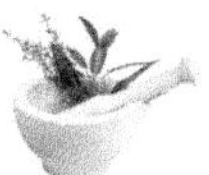

Cabbage Palm

Botanical Name:
Sabal palmetto

Family:
Arecaceae (**Palm family**)

Common Names:
Sabal palm, Palmetto palm, Cabbage palm • Manipuri: *Kona*

Description:
Cabbage palm is a beautiful and versatile palm, and is hence quite popular. It is recognised by its tan-gray, unbranched trunk, and large crown with fanlike leaves. The large leaves have a dull finish and are a medium green, sometimes yellow-green, in colour depending on the individual and

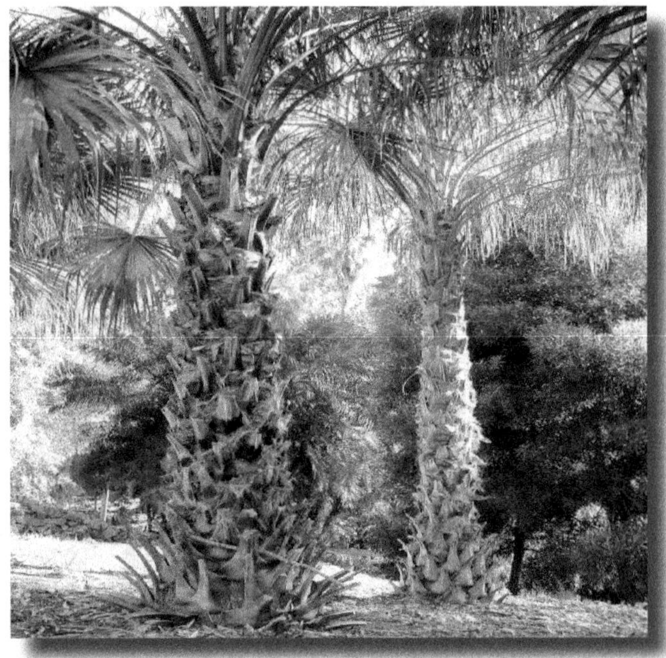

situation. Each leaf is up to 12 ft long overall including the *spineless petioles* (leaf stems) which measure about 5-6 ft in length. Leaves emerge directly from the trunk which is often covered with old leaf stem bases that are arranged in an interesting criss-cross pattern. Depending on the individual these may persist to the ground even in very old palms. Cabbage palm grows to a height of 10 - 25 m (32-82 feet), with a stem diameter of approximately 30 - 60 cm. In mid-summer the cabbage palm bears creamy white flowers on a long branched inflorescence that is held completely within the crown. Flowers are followed in late fall or early winter by black and fleshy spherical fruits that is about one-third of an inch in diameter.

Medicinal Uses:
Roots are cooling and restorative. The juice of a plant is *diuretic, stimulant, antiphlegmatic* and useful in *dropsy*. Cabbage palm is native to the *Americas*.

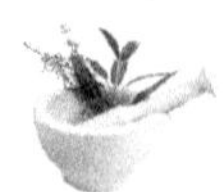

Green Milkweed Creeper

Botanical Name:

Cosmostigma racemosum

Family:

Asclepiadaceae (**Milkweed family**)

Synonyms:

Asclepias racemosa

Common Names:

Green Milkweed Creeper • Marathi: *Shendvel, Jati, Marvel* • Tamil: *Perum kahamugan kodi* • Malayalam: *Vattu valli* • Kannada: *Ghara hoovu gida*

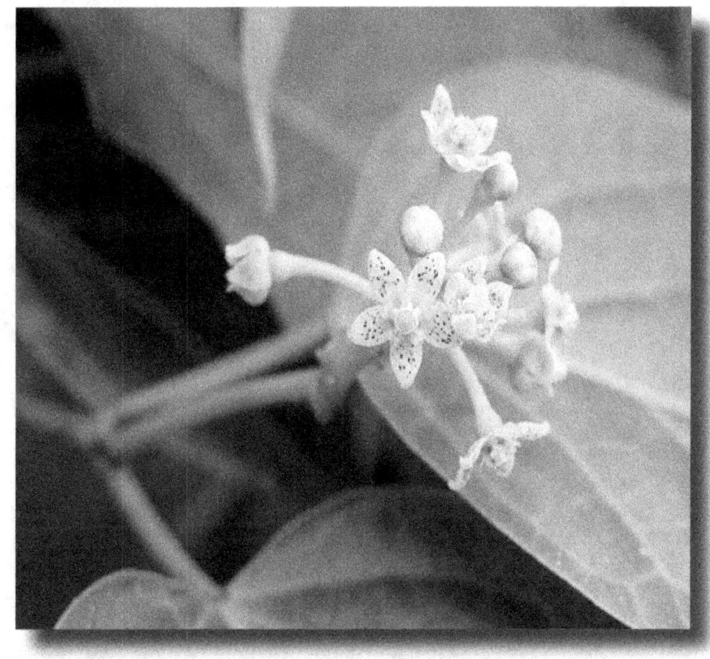

Description:

Green Milkweed Creeper is a twining shrub with watery sap. Stem are hollow within, sparsely hairy when young. Oppositely arranged leaves 7.5-11 x 3.5-5 cm, are broadly ovate, sharp tipped, with a rounded or heart-shaped base. Leaf stalks are 1.5-3 cm long. Small greenish flowers occur in corymb-like or raceme-like; peduncle 1.5-2.5 cm long. Sepals are 1.5 mm long, 5 in number. Flowers flat, wheel-like, 8-10 mm across, with 5 petals and very short tube. Petals are 4 mm long, ovate, yellowish-green with reddish-brown speckles. Stamens 5; filaments united; anthers 2-celled; Carpels 2, free ; style short, apex 5-angled. Flowering: July.

Medicinal Uses:

The leaves of this woody climber are used in *Indian traditional medicine* to cure *ulcerous sores*.

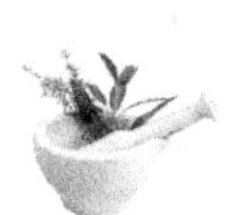

Gurmar

Botanical Name:

Gymnema sylvestre

Family:

Asclepiadaceae (**Milkweed family**)

Common Names:

Gurmar • Hindi: *Chhota-dudhilata, Gudmar, Gurmar, Medhashingi,* • Marathi: *Kavali, Bedaki, Bedakuli, Kalikardori, Kaoli* • Tamil: *Adigam, Amudupushpam, Ayagam, Kogilam* • Malayalam: *Chakkarakkolli, Madhunasini* • Telugu: *Bodaparta, Podapatra* • Kannada: *Kadhasige, Sannagera, Sannagerasehambu* • Oriya: *Meshasringi* • Urdu: *Gurmar, Gurmar booti, Gurmar patta* • Sanskrit: *Ajaballi, Ajaghandini, Karnika, Kshinavartta, Madhunasini*

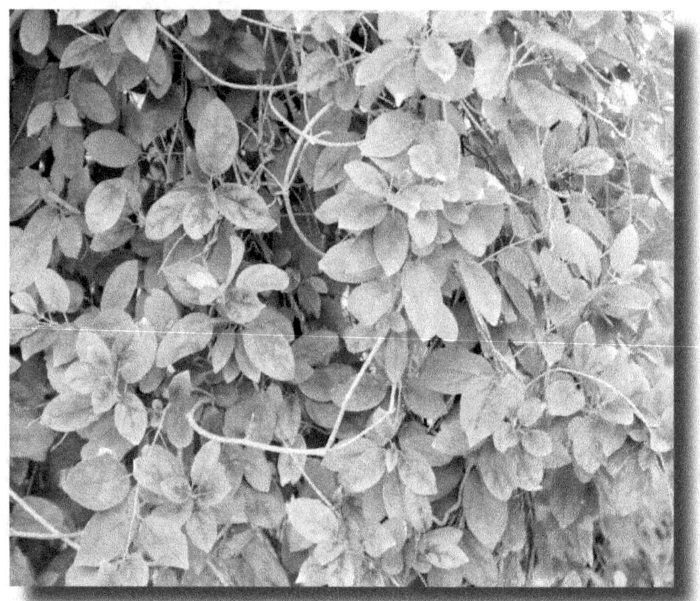

Description:

Gurmar is a famed plant, revered for its use in treatment of *diabetes* for nearly two millennia. The Hindi Name *Gurmar* actually means *diabetes killer*. It is a large climber, rooting at nodes. Leaves are elliptic, narrow tipped, and the base is narrow. Leaves are smooth above, and sparsely or densely velvety beneath. Pale yellow flowers are small, in axillary and lateral umbel like cymes. Stalk of the umbel is long. Sepals are long, ovate, obtuse and velvety. Flowers are pale yellow and bell-shaped. The corona is single, with five fleshy scales.

Medicinal Uses:

One of the alternative medicines to both *diabetes* and *obesity* could be *Gurmar plant preparation,* as it known to have a good effect for curbing of diabetes by blocking sugar binding sites and hence *not allowing the sugar molecules to accumulate in the body.*

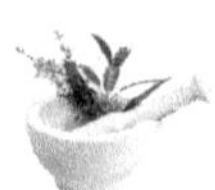

Indian Sarsaparilla

Botanical Name:
Hemidesmus indicus

Family:
Asclepiadaceae (**Milkweed family**)

Common Names:
Indian Sarsaparilla • Hindi: *Anantamul, Dudhli* • Manipuri: *Anantamul* • Marathi: *Anant vel* • Tamil: *Nannari, Sugandipala* • Malayalam: *Narunenti* • Telugu: *Suganda pala* • Kannada: *Sugankha-palada-gidda, Sogade* • Oriya: *Onotomulo* • Gujarati: *Sariva, Upalasari* • Sanskrit: *Anantamul, Sariva*

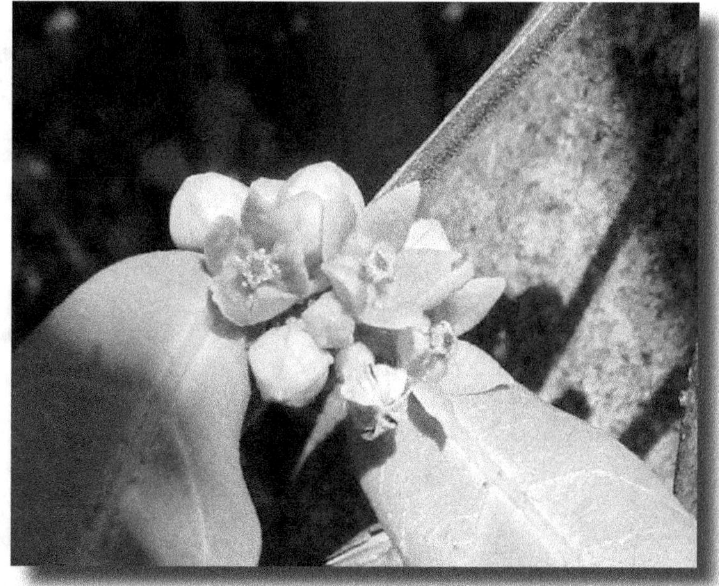

Description:
Indian Sarsaparilla is a vine, which trails on the ground and climbs by means of tendrils growing in pairs from the petioles of the alternate, orbicular to ovate, evergreen leaves. The vine emerges from a long, tuberous rootstock, and can reach up to 1-3 m. The Hindi name, *Anantamool* literally means, *endless root*. The small, greenish flowers grow in auxiliary umbels. The flower cymes are stalkless. Flowers have five petals, greenish on the outside and purple to yellowish orange on the inside. The flower petals are fleshy, typical of the Milkweed family to which it belongs. Now the Milkweed family has been incorporated in the Oleander family. Flowering: October-January.

Medicinal Uses:
It is one of the *Rasayana plants of Ayurveda*, as it is anabolic in its effect. It is used for *venereal diseases, herpes, skin diseases, arthritis, rheumatism, gout, epilepsy, insanity, chronic nervous diseases, abdominal distention, intestinal gas, debility, impotence* and *turbid urine*.

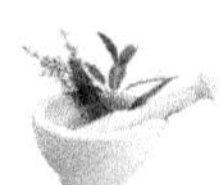

Holostemma Creeper

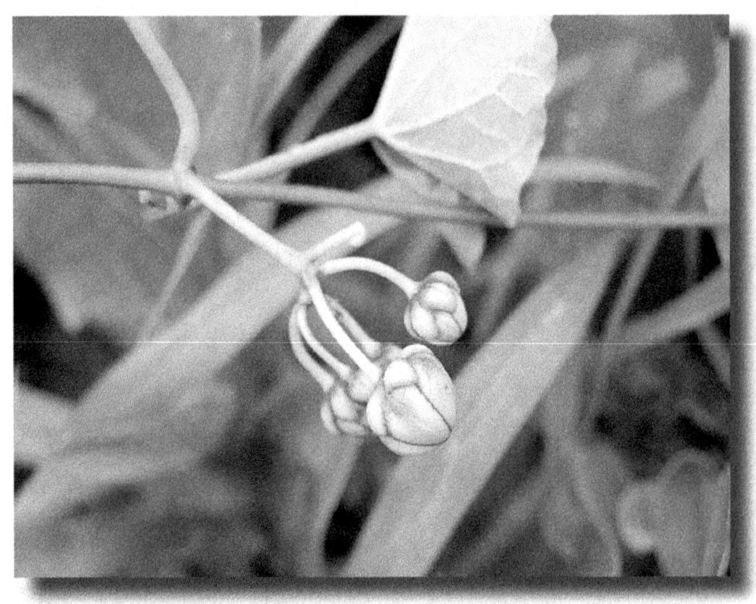

Botanical Name:

Holostemma ada-kodien

Family:

Asclepiadaceae (**Milkweed family**)

Synonyms:

Holostemma annulare

Common Names:

Holostemma Creeper • Hindi: *Chhirvel* • Marathi: *Dudruli, Shidodi* • Tamil: *Palay kirai* • Malayalam: *Ada kodien* • Telugu: *Palagurugu* • Sanskrit: *Jivanti, Arkapushpi*

Description:

Holostemma Creeper is a handsome, extensive, laticiferous, twining shrub with large conspicuous flowers. The bark is deeply cracked. The leaves are ovate to heart-shaped, 5-12 × 2-8 cm, coriaceous, acute, smooth above, and finely pubescent. The flowers are greenish-yellow in colour, purplish crimson inside, in lateral cymes. The petals are thick, typical of the milkweed family. Flowers are very fragrant. The central crown is edible. The fruits follicles sub-woody, 6-9 cm long, tapering and green. The roots are pretty long up to a meter or more in length, thick, cylindrical and irregularly twisted. It grows over hedges and in open forests especially on the lower slopes of hills. But its occurrence has diminished very much within this range of distribution and hence, it is considered endangered. Flowering: April-September.

Medicinal Uses:

Mainly the roots and the whole plant are used for medicinal purposes. Externally, the paste of its leaves and roots alleviate oedema due to vitiation of *pitta dosa*. The herb is beneficial for external use in various skin diseases, wounds and inflammation of the skin.

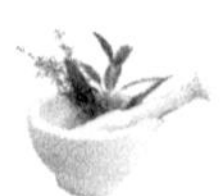

Pergularia

Botanical Name:
Pergularia daemia

Family:
Asclepiadaceae (**Milkweed family**)

Synonyms:
Asclepias daemia, Daemia extensa, Cynanchum extensum

Common Names:
Pergularia • Hindi: *Utaran, Sagovani, Aakasan, Gadaria Ki Bel, Jutak* • Marathi: *Utarn* • Tamil: *Uttamani, Seendhal kodi* • Malayalam: *Veliparatti* • Telugu: *Dustapuchettu, Jittupaku* • Kannada: *Halokoratige, Juttuve, Talavaranaballi, Bileehatthi balli* • Bengali: *Chagalbati, Ajashringi* • Oriya: *Utrali* • Sanskrit: *Uttamarani, Kurutakah, Visanika, Kakajangha*

Description:
Pergularia is a perennial twining herb, foul-smelling when bruised and with much milky juice, stem hairy. Leaves are thin, broadly ovate, heart-shaped or nearly circular, hairless above, velvety beneath. Greenish yellow or dull white, and sweet-scented flowers are borne in lateral cymes which are at first corymb-like, afterwards raceme-like. The five petals are hairy and spreading outwards. Corona outer and inner, outer truncate, inner curved high over the staminal column, spur acute. Fruit is a follicle, with soft spines all over and a long beak. Seeds are densely velvety on both sides. Flowering: August-February.

Medicinal Uses:
Pergularia has been used in *folk medicine* for the treatment of *liver disorders*.

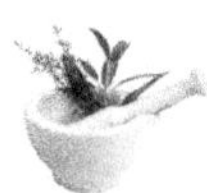

Indian Ipecac

Botanical Name:

Tylophora indica

Family:

Asclepiadaceae (**Milkweed family**)

Synonyms:

Asclepias asthmatica, Tylophora asthmatica, Cynanchum indicum

Common Names:

Indian Ipecac, Indian ipecacuahna • Hindi: *Antamul, Jangli pikvam* • Marathi: *Khadari, Pitthakaadi, Pitthamaari, Pitvel* • Tamil: *Naippalai, Nancaruppan* • Malayalam: *Nansjera-patsja, Vallippala* • Telugu: *Kakapala, Tellayadala, Verripala* • Kannada: *Antamula, Nipaladaberu, Aadumuttada gida* • Bengali: *Antamul* • Oriya: *Mendi, Mulini* • Assamese: *Antamul* • Sanskrit: *Arkaparni, Lataksiri, Shwasaghni*

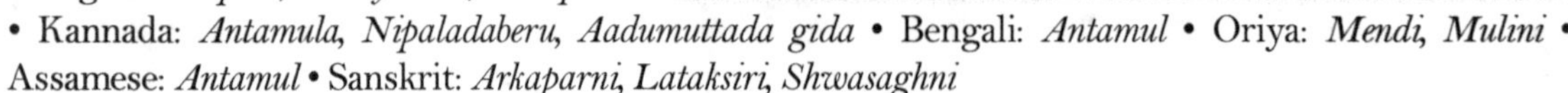

Description:

Indian Ipecac is a small, slender, much branched, velvety, twining or climbing herb with yellowish sap. It is mostly found in the sub-Himalayan tract from Uttarakhand to Meghalaya and in the central and peninsular India. Rootstock is 2.5-5 cm, thick. Leaves, 6-11 cm long, 3.8-6 cm wide, are ovate-oblong to elliptic-oblong, with a narrow tip, heart-shaped at base, thick, velvety beneath when young, and smooth above. Leaf stalks are up to 1.2 cm long. Flowers are small, 1-1.5 cm across, in 2 to 3-flowered fascicles in cymes in leaf axils. Sepal up is divided nearly to the base, and densely hairy outside. Sepals are lance-shaped. Flowers are greenish- yellow or greenish-purple, with oblong, pointy, petals. *The fruit is a follicle,* up to 7 x 1 cm, ovoid-lance-shaped. Flowering: August-December.

Medicinal Uses:

It is traditionally used as a *folk remedy* in certain regions of India for the treatment of *bronchial asthma, inflammation, bronchitis, allergies, rheumatism and dermatitis.*

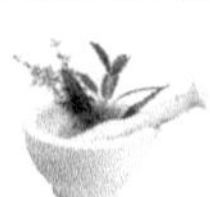

Aloe Vera

Botanical Name:

Aloe vera

Family:

Asphodelaceae (**Aloe family**)

Synonyms:

Aloe barbadensis, Aloe indica, Aloe vulgaris

Common Names:

Aloe vera, Medicinal aloe, Burn plant • Hindi: *Gheekumari* • Marathi: *Khorpad* • Tamil: *Kathalai* • Malayalam: *Chotthu kathalai*

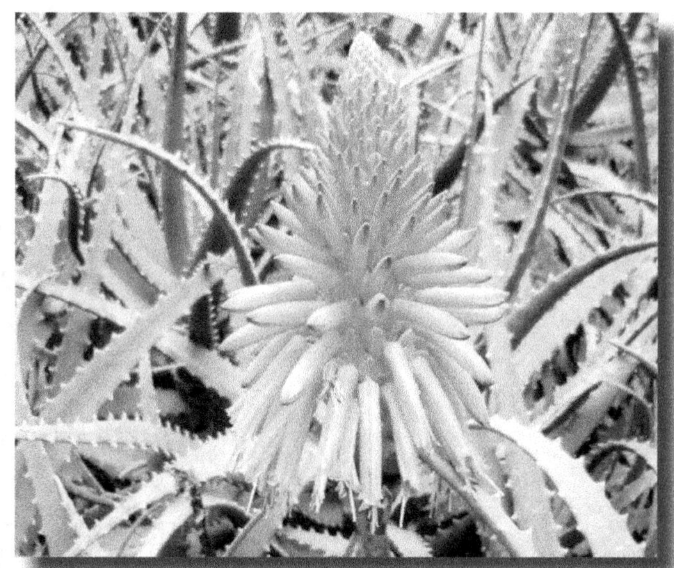

Description:

Aloe, a popular houseplant, has a long history as a multipurpose folk remedy. Commonly known as Aloe vera, the plant can be snapped off and placed on cuts and burns for immediate relief. Aloe vera is a clump forming succulent whose fleshy gray-green leaves are arranged in a vase shaped rosette atop a very short stem. The leaves are up to 18 in long and 2 in wide at the base, slightly grooved on top, and terminating in a sharp point. The leaves have small grayish teeth on the margins. The main rosette gets up to about 2 ft high, and the plant continually produces little offset rosettes. In winter and spring, medicinal aloe bears small tubular yellow flowers on branched stalks up to 3 ft tall. The real Aloe vera has yellow flowers, but many of the clones available have orange flowers. Although Aloe Vera is a member of the Lily family, it is very-cactus like in its characteristics.

Medicinal Uses:

Aloe Vera contains *over 20 minerals*, all of which are essential to the human body. The human body requires 22 amino acids for good health — eight of which are called "essential" because the body cannot fabricate them. Aloe Vera contains all of these eight essential amino acids, and 11 of the 14 "secondary" amino acids. Aloe Vera has Vitamins A, B1, B2, B6, B12, C and E. In India, Aloe vera is believed to help in sustaining youth, due to its positive effects on the skin. Hence, it is called *ghee kunvar* or *ghee kumaari*.

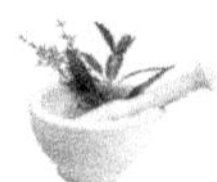

Common Yarrow

Botanical Name:

Achillea millefolium

Family:

Asteraceae (**Sunflower family**)

Synonyms:

Achillea lanulosa, Achillea magna

Common Names:

Common Yarrow, Sneezewort, Soldier's friend, Thousand-leaf • Hindi: *Gandrain, Puthkanda, Bhut Kesi* • Marathi: *Rojmaari* • Tamil: *Achchilliya* • Konkani: *Rajmari* • Urdu: *Tukhm gandana, Buiranjasif, Brinjasuf*

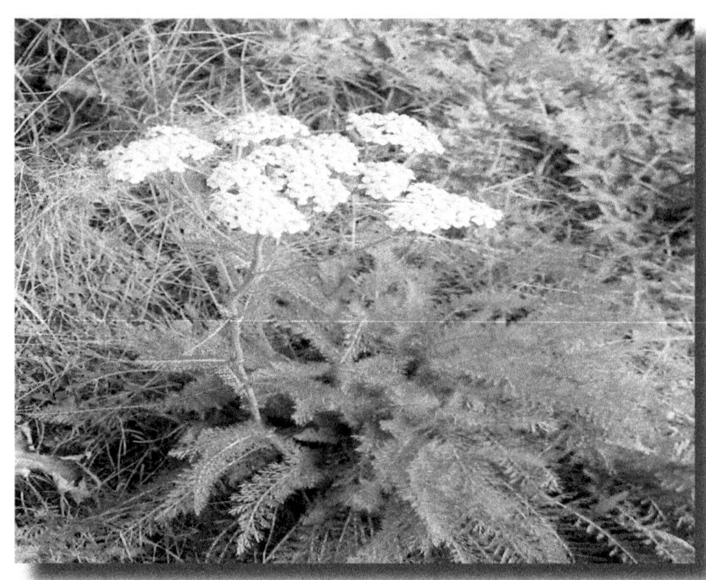

Description:

Yarrows are herbaceous perennials, most with fragrant lacy foliage and small daisy-like flowerheads borne in rounded corymbs. Common yarrow has leaves that are grayish green, aromatic, and very finely dissected, like soft dainty ferns. The plant forms dense spreading mats of lacy leaves from rhizomes that creep beneath the ground surface. In summer yarrow sends up erect, grayish, usually unbranched stems, 1-3 ft tall. The fifty or more small, about 0.25 in across with whitish flowerheads are borne in flat to domed clusters. Flower have white, 5-ray petals that surround tiny yellow to light cream-coloured disc florets, each flower head is 3-5 mm across; occur as independent and terminal round or flat-topped clusters; clusters are 6-30 cm across. The plant may have been Named after the Greek person Achilles. Within India, Common Yarrow is found in the Himalayan region of Jammu & Kashmir, Himachal Pradesh, Uttarakhand in an altitude range of 1050-3600 m.

Medicinal Uses:

In *Greek mythology*, it is said to have been used by *Achilles* to heal his warriors during the battle of Troy - hence the Name 'Achillea'. In *Anglo-Saxon times, it was used as a charm to ward off evil and illness* - and as a treatment for wounds, much as Achilles used it, giving it a common Name for the period of 'Soldier's Wound-Wort'. Yarrow has been used to stop bleeding by inserting leaves into the nostrils of wounded soldiers. Druids used Yarrow to predict seasonal weather. *In Chinese legends, Yarrow was used to predict the future.*

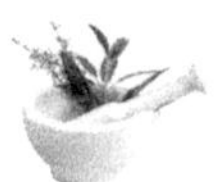

Toothache Plant

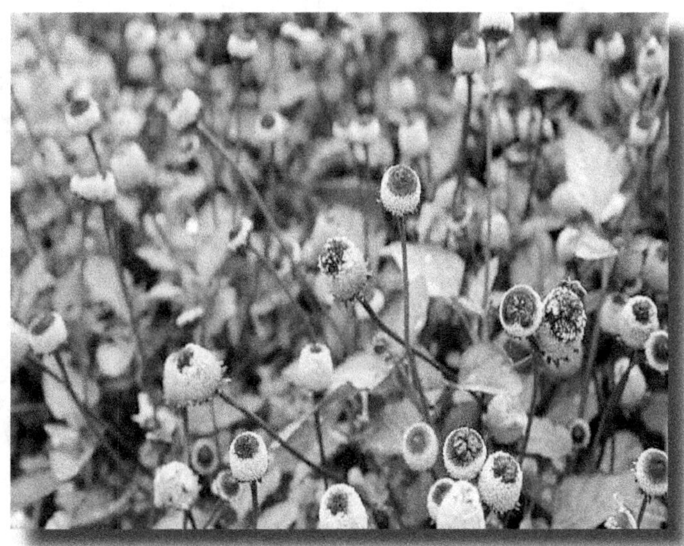

Botanical Name:
Acmella oleracea

Family:
Asteraceae **(Sunflower family)**

Synonyms:
Spilanthes acmella, Spilanthes oleracea

Common Names:
Toothache Plant, Para cress • Hindi: *Akarkar, Pipulka* • Marathi: *Pipulka, Akarkara* • Kannada: *Hemmugalu* • Assamese: *Pirazha*

Description:
Toothache Plant or 'Paracress' is a flowering herb. Its leaves and flower heads contain an analgesic agent that may be used to numb toothaches. It is grown as an orNamental (and occasionally as a medicinal) in various parts of the world. The stems are prostrate or erect, often reddish, hairless. Leaves are broadly ovate to triangular, 5–11 cm long, 4–8 cm wide, margins toothed, tip sharp. Flower-heads arise singly, elongated-conical, containing primarily disc florets, 1–2.4 cm long, 1.1–1.7 cm in diameter. Disc florets are many, yellow to orange, 2.7–3.3 mm long. Achenes are black, 2–2.5 mm long. Eating Toothache Plant is a memorable experience. The leaf has a smell similar to any green leafy vegetable. The taste, however, is somewhat reminiscent of Echinacea, but lacking the bitter and sometimes nauseating element of that medicinal. First, a strong, spicy warmth spreads outward across one's tongue, turning into a prickling sensation. With this the salivary glands leap into action, pumping out quantities of saliva. As the prickling spreads, it mellows into an acidic (slightly metallic) sharpness accompanied by tingling, and then numbness. The numbness fades after a time (two to twenty minutes, depending on the person and amount eaten), and the pungent aftertaste may linger for an hour or more.

Medicinal Uses:
The leaves and flower heads contain *analgesic, antifungal, anthelminthic* and *antibacterial* agents, but some of the compounds are destroyed by *desiccation or freezing.*

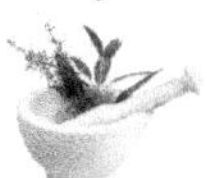

Sticky Daisy

Botanical Name:

Adenostemma lavenia

Family:

Asteraceae (**Sunflower family**)

Synonyms:

Verbesina lavenia, Adenostemma viscosum

Common Names:

Sticky Daisy, Clubwort, • Hindi: *Jangli-jira* • Konkani: *Ghanerem*

Description:

Sticky Daisy is a native species found in open, wet places along streams, in forest and in thickets, from sea level to an altitude of 1,800 metres. It is an erect, smooth

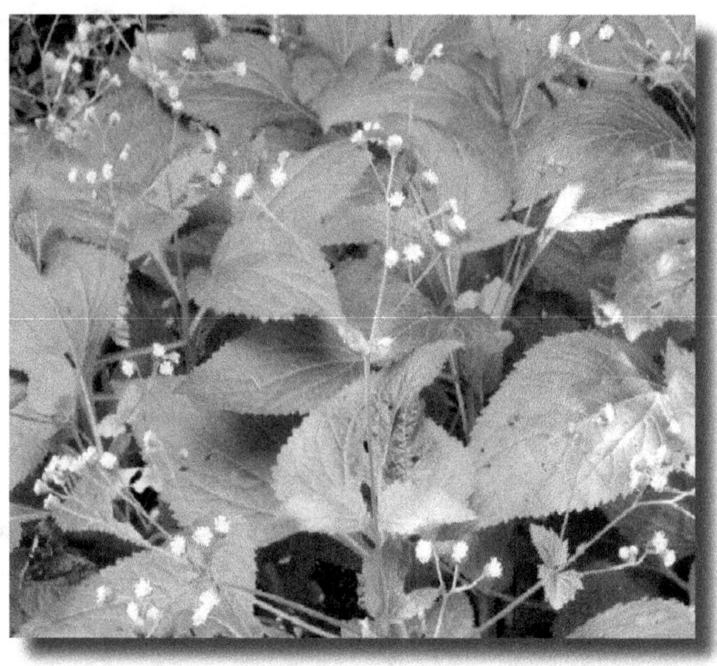

or hairy, annual, slender or rather stout herb 0.3-1 m in height. The leaves are thin, opposite (upper ones alternate), oblong to broadly ovate, and 5-15 cm long, with the apex pointed and the margins entire or scalloped. The inflorescence is lax, and the heads are 5-7 mm in diameter. The flowers are very small and white, with the corolla hairy near the mouth. The achene is covered with wrinkles or is rough, and is crowned by a glandular ring bearing 3 to 5 club-shaped, short lobes.

Medicinal Uses:

The plant is used in *medicine worldwide*. In India, the *extract of leaves is applied to injuries.*

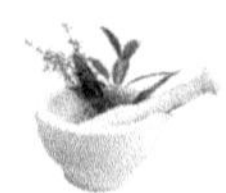

Goat Weed

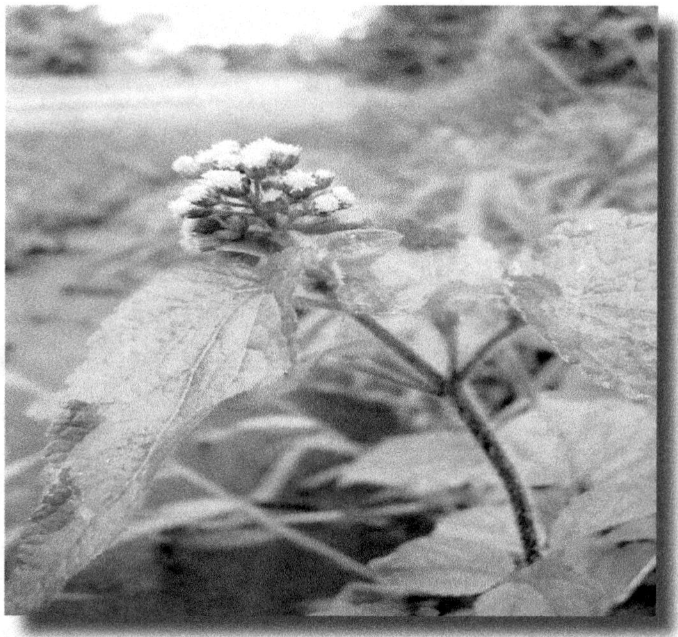

Botanical Name:

Ageratum conyzoides

Family:

Asteraceae (**Sunflower family**)

Common Names:

Goat weed, Billy goat weed, Tropical whiteweed • Hindi: *Jangli pudina, Visadodi, Semandulu, Gha buti, Bhakumbar* • Manipuri: *Khongjai napi* • Marathi: *Ghanera osaadi* • Kannada: *Oorala gida, Helukasa* • Tamil: *Pumppillu, Appakkoti* • Malayalam: *Kattappa, Muriyan pacca* • Bengali: *Uchunti* • Sanskrit: *Visamustih*

Description:

Goat weed is a common tropical annual herbaceous weed. It is an erect softly hairy annual plant which grows up to a height of 2.5 feet. Oppositely arranged leaves are ovate to lance-like, coarsely rounded, and have toothed margin. Numerous pale blue or whitish flowerheads are 6 mm across, often forming dense domed to flat-topped clusters in leaf axils or end of branches. Flowers most of the year. The stem is often red and has long white hairs. The weak aromatic unpleasant smelling leaves are also covered with fine hair. The dark seeds have scales and ends in a needle-like shape.

Medicinal Uses:

In alternative medicine, ageratum is used against *epilepsy and wounds*, also used as an *insect repellent*.

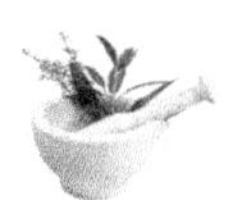

Indian Wormwood

Botanical Name:
Artemisia nilagirica

Family:
Asteraceae (**Sunflower family**)

Synonyms:
Artemisia vulgaris, Artemisia vulgaris var. nilagirica

Common Names:
Indian Wormwood, Fleabane, Mugwort • Hindi: *Nagdona, Davana* • Manipuri: *Leibakngou* • Marathi: *Dhordavana, Gondhomaro* • Tamil: *Makkippu* • Malayalam: *Makkippuvu, Masipatri* • Telugu: *Masipatri* • Kannada: *Manjepatre, Urigattige* • Bengali: *Nagadana* • Oriya: *Dayona* • Konkani: *Surpin* • Assamese: *Nilum* • Sanskrit: *Nagadaman, Damanak*

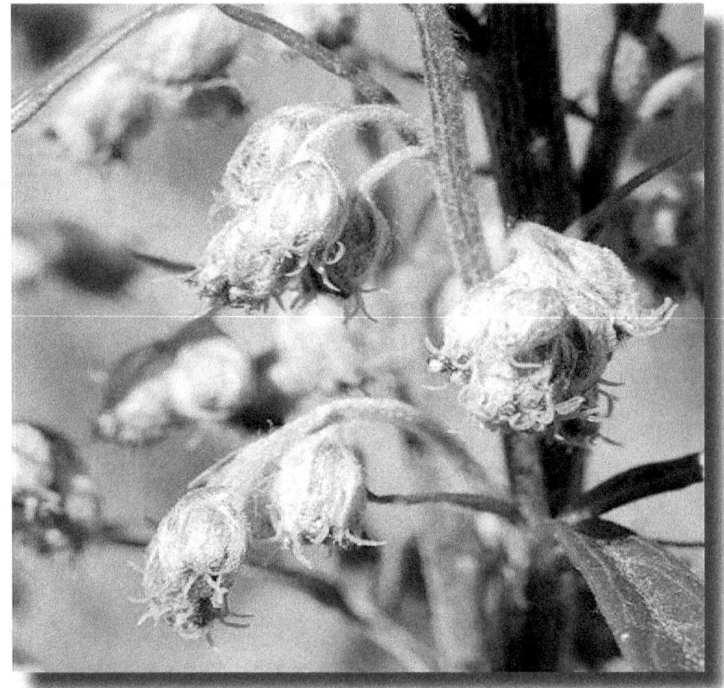

Description:
Indian Wormwood is an *aromatic shrub*, 1-2 m high, with yellow or dark red small flowers, and grows throughout India in *hills up to 2400 m elevation*. This medicinal herb is erect, hairy, often half-woody. The stems are leafy and branched. The leaves are pinnately lobed, 5-14 cm long, grey beneath. The Mugwort blossoms with reddish brown or yellow flowers. The flowers are freely small and stand in long narrow clusters at the top of the stem. The fruit (achene) is minute. It is believed that Indian Wormwood drives away insects. So the leaves and flowers are put in boxes and cupboards.

Medicinal Uses:
In Manipur, the leaves are used to prepare a local hair-care lotion, *Chinghi*.

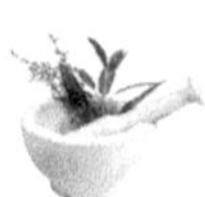

Spanish Needles

Botanical Name:

Bidens biternata

Family:

Asteraceae (**Sunflower family**)

Synonyms:

Coreopsis biternata

Common Names:

Spanish Needles, Yellow flowered blackjack, Black jack, Five leaved blackjack, Beggar ticks • Hindi: *Chirchitta*

Description:

Spanish Needles is an erect annual herb, up to 1 m. Closely related to B. pilosa, but can be distinguished by

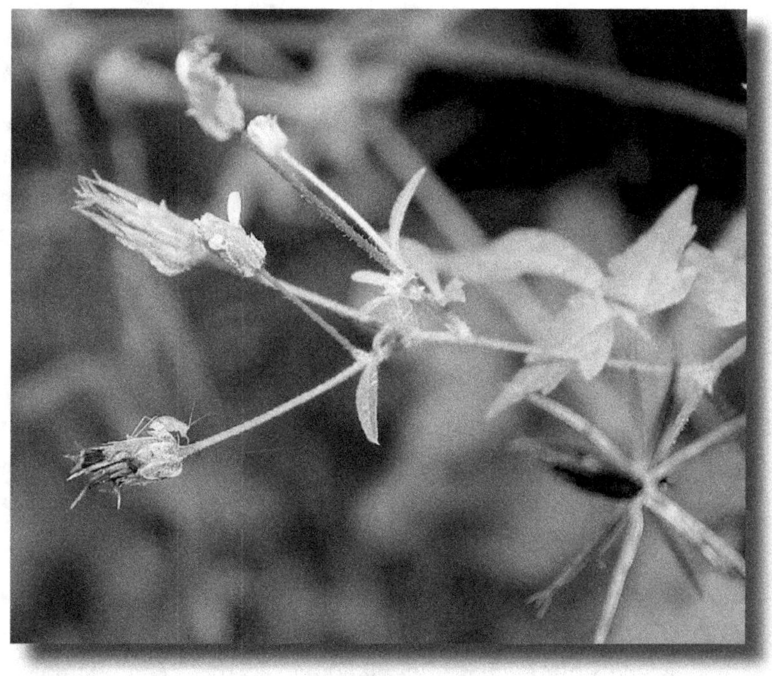

the leaves, which are usually 5-7 foliolate, with the lowermost pair redivided into two to three segments. The outer involucral bracts resemble those of B. bipinnata. The achenes are up to 16 mm long, almost glabrous. The flowers are yellow, including the ray-florets. Spanish Needles is a widespread weed of disturbed and cultivated areas.

Medicinal Uses:

Used to treat *eye and ear affections* (leaf juice); applied to *skin affections* in general, as a *haemostatic on wounds*, and *wrapped around the umbilical cord of babies* (rubbed leaves).

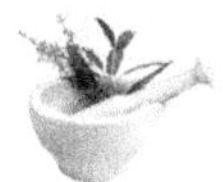

Kakronda

Botanical Name:

Blumea lacera

Family:

Asteraceae (**Sunflower family**)

Common Names:

Kakronda, Blumea • Hindi: *Jangli Muli, Kakronda* • Marathi: *Bhamurda, Burando* • Tamil: *Kattumullangi, Narakkarandai* • Telugu: *Advimulangi, Karupogaku* • Bengali: *Kukurmuta, Kukursunga* • Gujarati: *Kolhar, Pilo Kapurio* • Sanskrit: *Kukkuradru, Kukundara, Mridu chhada, Tamrachuda*

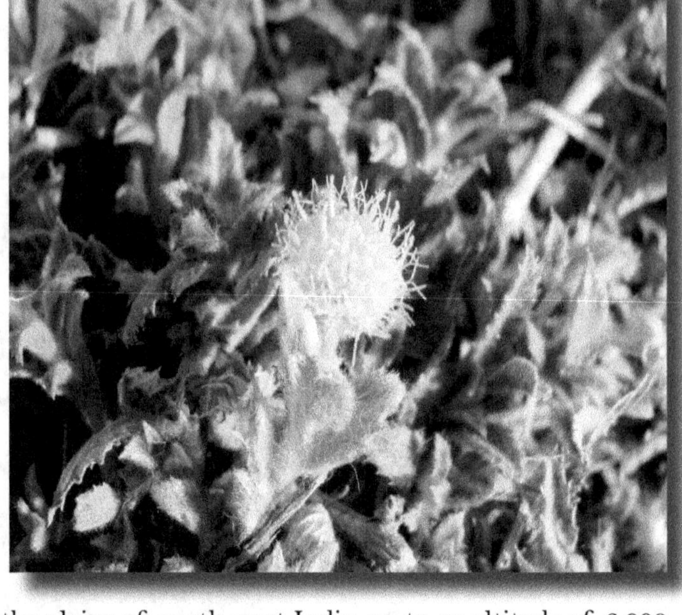

Description:

Kakronda is an *annual herb* with a strong odour, distributed throughout the plains of north-west India, up to an altitude of 2,000 m. The stems of this hairy or glandular herb are erect, simple or branched, very leafy and 1-2 ft in height. The leaves are obovate or oblanceolate, 5-12 cm long, 2-6 cm wide, smaller toward the top, stalked, and toothed or (rarely) lobulated at the margins. The bright yellow flowering heads are about 8 mm across, borne on short axillary cymes, and collected in terminal, spike-like panicles. The involucre-bracts are narrow and hairy. The achenes are not ribbed, and are somewhat 4-angled, and smooth.

Medicinal Uses:

Blumea is described by *Ayurveda experts as hot, pungent* and *bitter; antipyretic;* good for *bronchitis,* diseases of the *blood, fevers, thirst and burning sensations.* The root kept in the mouth is said to cure the diseases of the mouth. In the Konkan region of India, the plant is used to *drive away fleas and other insects.* In Homoeopathic system, it is given in *enuresis, neuralgia, headaches* and *cold borne cough.*

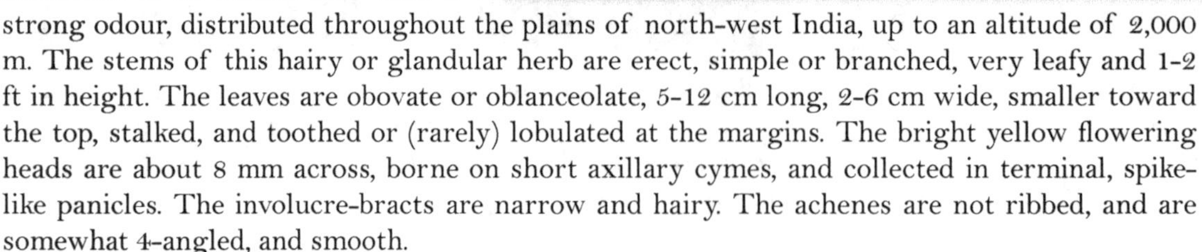

Safflower

Botanical Name:

Carthamus tinctorius

Family:

Asteraceae **(Sunflower family)**

Common Names:

Safflower, Dyers' saffron, False saffron • Hindi: *Kusum* • Manipuri: *Kusumlei* • Tamil: *Kusumba* • Urdu: *Gul rang*

Description:

Safflower is an annual plant native to the Mediterranean countries and cultivated in Europe and the U.S. Its glabrous, branching stem grows from 1

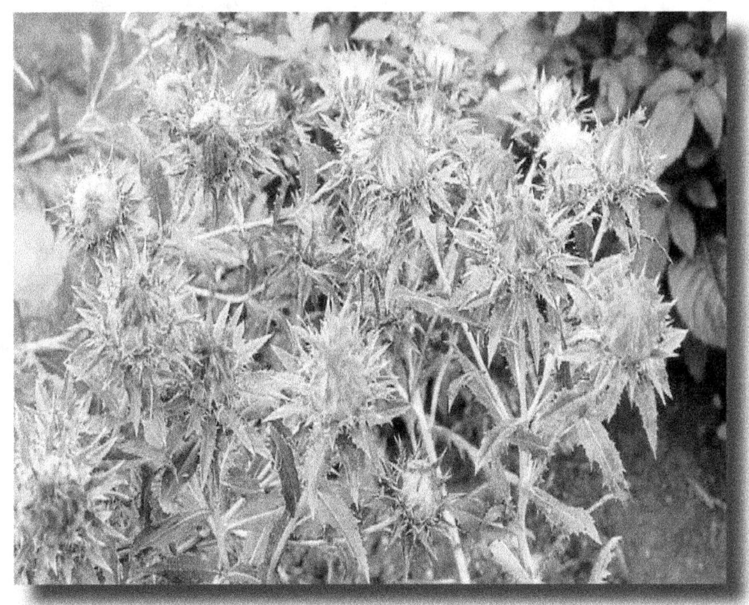

to 3 feet high and bears alternate, sessile, oblong, or ovate-lanceolate leaves armed with small, spiny teeth. The orange-yellow flowers grow in flower heads about 1 to 11/2 inches across. This thistle is valued for its orange-yellow flowers in summer and for the oil contained in its seeds. The orange-red flowers of safflower sometimes serve as a substitute for saffron, since they give a (rather pale) colour to the food. They are frequently sold as "saffron" to tourists in Hungary or Northern Africa (and probably many other parts of the world). Their value as spice is nearly nil, but their staining capability justifies usage in the kitchen.

Medicinal Uses:

Taken hot, safflower tea produces strong perspiration and has thus been used for colds and related ailments. It has also been used at times for its soothing effect in cases of *hysteria*, such as that associated with *chlorosis. Powdered seeds made into a poultice* is used to ally *inflammation* of *the womb* after *child birth. Flowers* of this herb is useful for *jaundice.*

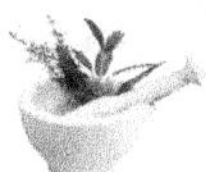

Siam Weed

Botanical Name:

Chromolaena odorata

Family:

Asteraceae (**Sunflower family**)

Synonyms:

Eupatorium odoratum

Common Names:

Siam Weed, Bitter bush, Devilweed, Hagonoy, Jack in the bush, Triffid weed • Hindi: Tivra gandha, Bagh dhoka • Malayalam: Communist Pacha, Venapacha

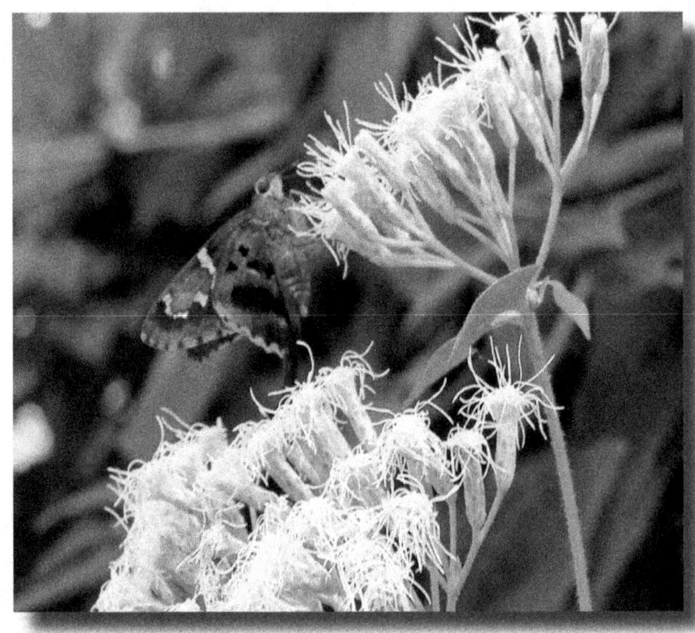

Description:

Siam Weed is a big bushy herb or subshrub with long rambling (but not twining branches. In open areas it spreads into tangled, dense thickets up to 2 m tall, and higher when climbing up vegetation. Many paired branches grow off the main stem. The base of the plant becomes hard and woody while the branch tips are soft and green. The leaves are arrowhead-shaped, 5–12 cm long and 3–7 cm wide, with three characteristic veins in a 'pitchfork' pattern. They grow in opposite pairs along the stems and branches. As the species Name 'odorata' suggests, the leaves emit a pungent odour when crushed. Clusters of 10–35 pale pink–mauve or white tubular flowers, 10 mm long, are found at the ends of branches. The seeds are dark coloured, 4–5 mm long, narrow and oblong, with a parachute of white hairs which turn brown as the seed dries. Siam weed is native to Tropical America, but is now naturalised throughout the tropics.

Medicinal Uses:

It is used as a *traditional medicine in Indonesia*. The *young leaves are crushed*, and the *resulting liquid* can be used to *treat skin wounds*.

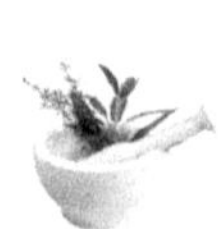

Chicory

Botanical Name:

Cichorium intybus

Family:

Asteraceae (**Sunflower family**)

Common Names:

Chicory, Blue sailors, Succory, Coffeeweed • Hindi: Kasni, Hinduba • Marathi: Kachani • Malayalam: Chikkari • Telugu: Kasini, Kasini-vittulu • Kannada: Chikory • Urdu: Kasni, Tukme-e-kasni, Barg-e-kasni • Sanskrit: Kasni

Description:

Chicory is a bushy perennial herb with blue or lavender flowers. It is a bushy perennial plant that attains a

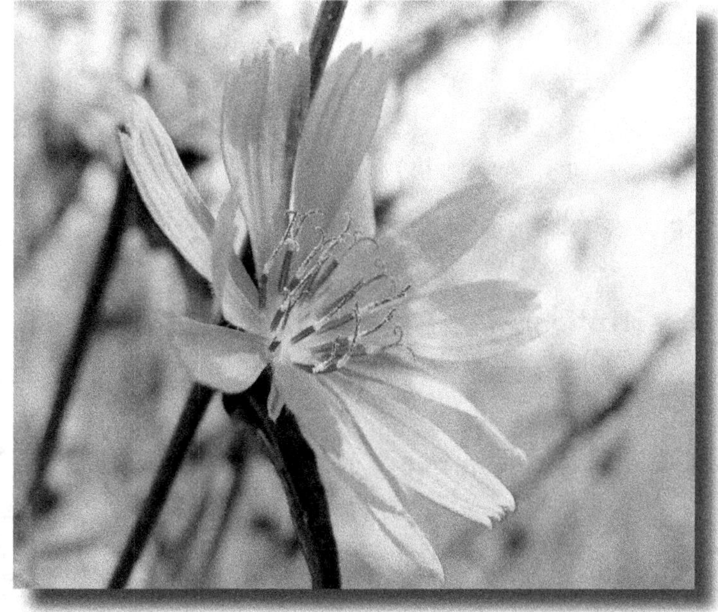

height of 1 to 4 feet. The stem has edges having hard branches. Flowers occur either solitary on nearly leafless branches, or in clusters in leaf axils. Flower-heads are 2.5-4 cm across, with spreading ray-florets. The green bracts below the flowers are prominent. The outer lancelike bracts are spreading outwards, while the longer inner ones are upright. Leaves are oblong-lancelike, and lower leaves are pinnately lobed. The upper leaves are entire, bract-like, stem-clasping. Root is like a tail of a cow and is fleshy having brownish colour from outside and white colour from inside. It has a length of 2 ½ feet and has a bitter taste. Chicory is grown for its leaves, or for the roots, which are baked, ground, and used as a coffee substitute in instant coffee. In India Chicory is found in the northwestern regions like Kashmir and Punjab and in areas of south India.

Medicinal Uses:

The ancient Egyptians ate large amounts of chicory because it was believed that the plant could *purify the blood and liver,* while others have relied on the herb for its power to cure 'passions of the heart.' *Chicory continues to be a popular herbal remedy due to its healing effects on several ailments.*

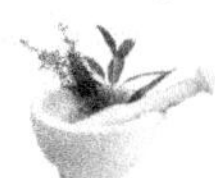

Wild Cosmos

Botanical Name:

Cosmos caudatus

Family:

Asteraceae **(Sunflower family)**

Common Names:

Wild Cosmos, Ulam Raja

Description:

Wild Cosmos is a wild cousin of the popular garden plant, Cosmos. It is an annual herb, growing 1–8 ft tall, hairless or sparsely hairy. Leaf stalks are 1–7 cm long. Leaves are finely dissected, 10–20 cm long.

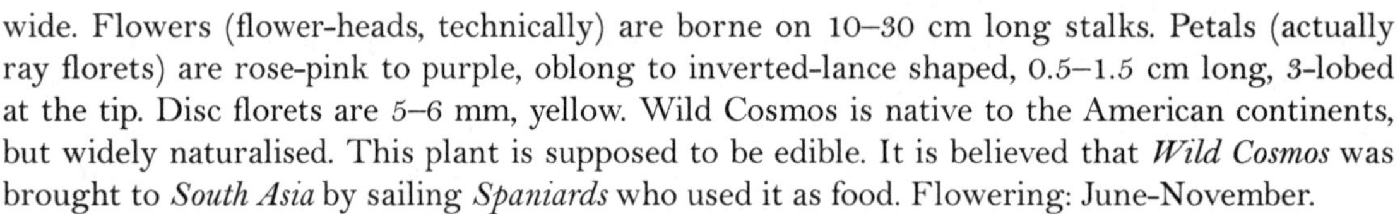

Ultimate lobes are 2–10 mm wide. Flowers (flower-heads, technically) are borne on 10–30 cm long stalks. Petals (actually ray florets) are rose-pink to purple, oblong to inverted-lance shaped, 0.5–1.5 cm long, 3-lobed at the tip. Disc florets are 5–6 mm, yellow. Wild Cosmos is native to the American continents, but widely naturalised. This plant is supposed to be edible. It is believed that *Wild Cosmos* was brought to *South Asia* by sailing *Spaniards* who used it as food. Flowering: June-November.

Medicinal Uses:

In South-east Asia, the plant is used traditionally for improving blood circulation.

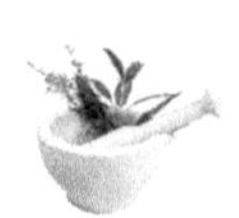

Thickhead

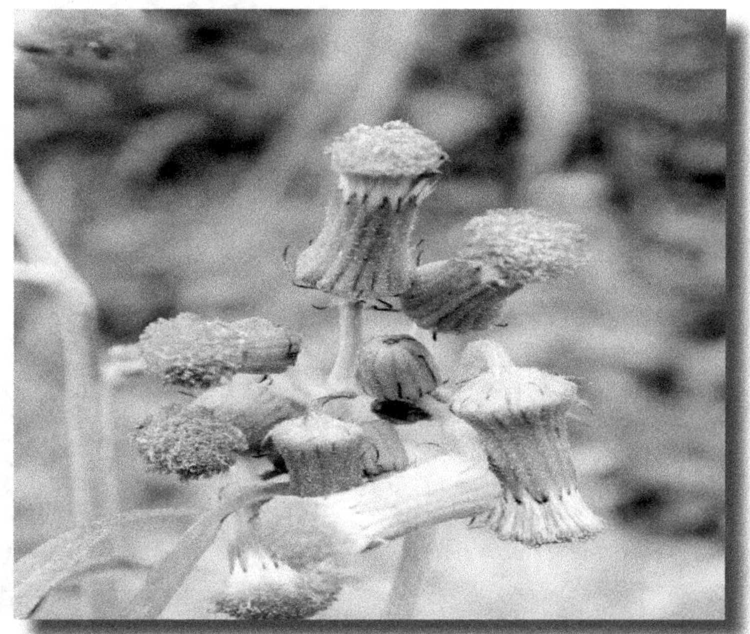

Botanical Name:

Crassocephalum crepidioides

Family:

Asteraceae **(Sunflower family)**

Synonyms:

Gynura crepidioides

Common Names:

Thickhead, Fireweed, Redflower ragleaf • Manipuri: Tera paibi

Description:

Fireweed is an erect little-branched herb to 1 m tall, smooth or finely hairy. Leaves with lamina elliptic to ovate in outline; lowest leaves lyrate-pinnatifid, up to 20 cm long and 10 cm wide, base often with a pair of stipule-like lobes, margins coarsely toothed; upper leaves smaller, not lobed or with a lobe each side towards base; petiole up to 4 cm long.

Heads in cymes, few to many, nodding at first, later erect; heads 4 mm diameter. Flowerheads are cylindrical, green, with red florets visible on top. Seeds are floating balls of numerous silky white hair, which kids in India call by Names equivalent to 'old lady' in different languages. Thickhead is native to tropical Africa, but now naturalized in India and South-east Asia.

Medicinal Uses:

Its fleshy, mucilaginous leaves and stems are eaten as a vegetable. *A lotion of leaves* is used as a *mild medicine* that strengthens the *stomach* and *excites its actions.*

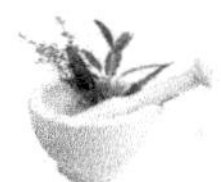

False Daisy

Botanical Name:

Eclipta prostrata

Family:

Asteraceae (**Sunflower family**)

Synonyms:

Eclipta erecta, Eclipta alba, Eclipta punctata, Verbesina prostrate

Common Names:

False Daisy, Trailing eclipta •Hindi: *Bhringaraj, Kesharaj* •Manipuri: *Uchi-sumbal* •Tamil: *Karisilanganni, Kavanthakara* • Malayalam: *Kannunni* •Telugu:*Galagara* •Kannada: *Ajagara* •Oriya: *Kesarda* •Sanskrit: *Bhringaraj*

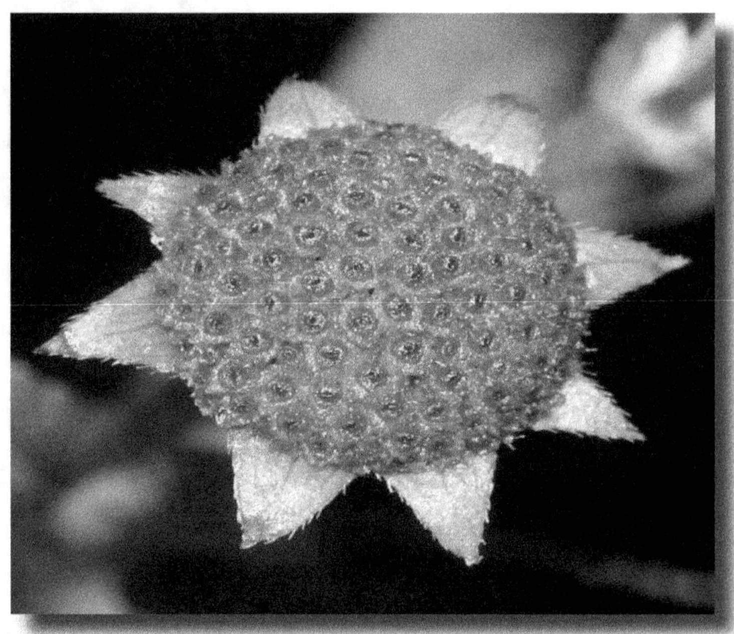

Description:

False Daisy is an annual commonly found growing in waste ground. Stems are erect or prostate, entirely velvety, often rooting at nodes. Oppositely arranged stalkless, oblong, lance-shaped, or elliptic leaves are 2.5-7.5 cm long. It has a short, flat or round, brown stem and small white daisy-like flowers on a long stalk. Eclipta grows abundantly in the tropics and is used with success in Ayurvedic medicine. Bhringaraj was used by Hindus in their Shradh, the ceremony for paying respect to a recently deceased person. This plant is one of the Hindu's "Ten Auspicious Flowers" and is sometimes called, "the king of hair."

Medicinal Uses:

Bhringraj is mainly used in hair oils, but it has been considered a good drug in hepatotoxicity. In *hair oils*, it may be used along with Centela asiatica (Brahmi) and Phyllanthus emblica (Amla) It may be used to prevent habitual abortion and miscarriage and also in cases of post-delivery uterine pain. A decoction of leaves is used in uterine haemorrhage. The juice of the plant with honey is given to infants with castor oil for expulsion of worms. For the relief in piles, fumigation with Eclipta alba is considered beneficial. The paste prepared by mincing fresh plants has got an anti-inflammatory effect and may be applied to *insect bites, stings, swellings* and other *skin diseases.*

Elephant Foot

Botanical Name:

Elephantopus scaber

Family:

Asteraceae (**Sunflower family**)

Common Names:

Elephant Foot, Prickly-leaved elephant's foot, Bull's Tongue, Ironweed • Hindi: *Samdudri, Bantambakhu* • Marathi: *Hastipata* • Tamil: *Anashovadi* • Malayalam: *Anayatiyan* • Telugu: *Enugabira* • Kannada: *Hakkarike* • Bengali: *Hasti pod* • Sanskrit: *Gojivha*

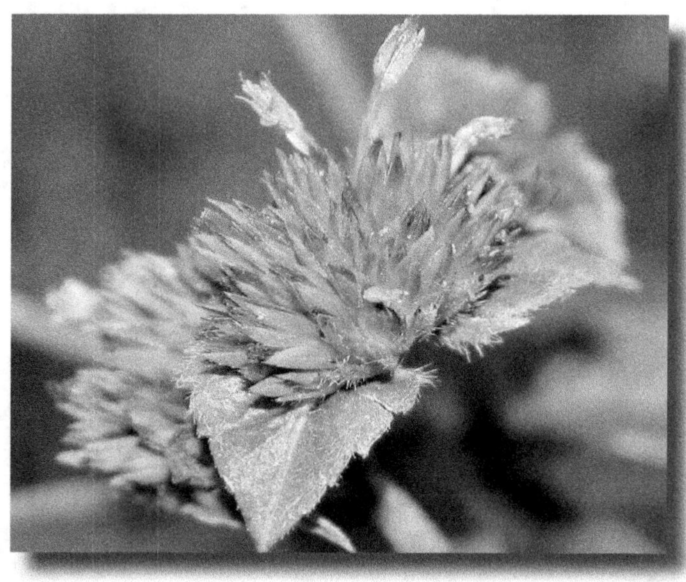

Description:

Elephant Foot is a rather coarse, rigid, erect, hairy herb 30 to 60 cm high. Stems forked, and stiff. Leaves are mostly in basal rosette and oblong-ovate to oblong-lancelike, 10-25 cm in length and often very much notched on the margins. Those on the stem few and much smaller. Purple flowers are 8-10 mm long. Each head comprises about 4 flowers. Flowering heads borne in clusters at the end of the branches and usually enclosed by 3 leaf-like bracts which are ovate to oblong-ovate, 1 to 1.5 cm long, and heart-shaped at the base. The flowering heads many-crowded in each cluster. Fruits are achenes, ribbed. Pappus from 4 to 6 mm long with rigid bristles.

Medicinal Uses:

Roots and leaves are used as *emollient for dysuria, diarrhoea, dysentery, swellings* and *stomach pain.* The *root* is prescribed to *prevent vomiting. Powdered with pepper, it is applied for toothaches. Leaves* are used in applications for *eczema* and *ulcers.*

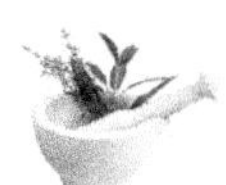

Burma Agrimony

Botanical Name:
Eupatorium birmanicum

Family:
Asteraceae (**Sunflower family**)

Common Names:
Burma Agrimony • Manipuri: *Langthrei*

Description:

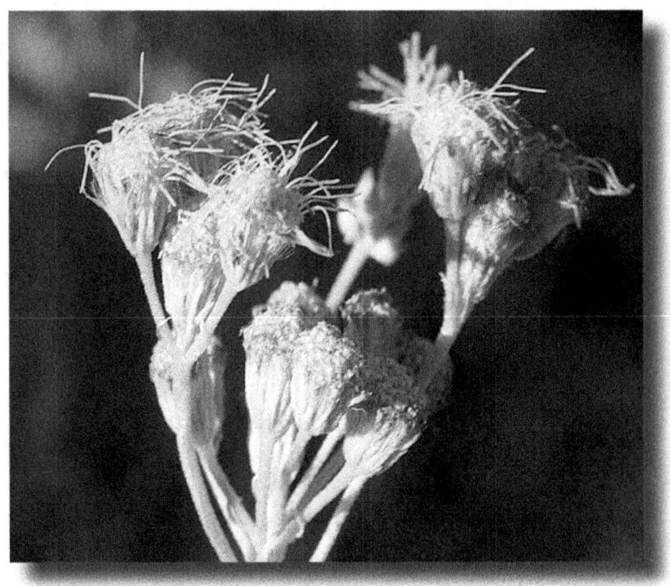

Eupatorium is a genus of flowering plants, which are herbaceous perennial plants growing to 0.5–3 m tall. Many of them are used in folk medicine, like the famed *Communist pacha* of Kerala. Burma Agrimony is a herb commonly found in North-East India, particularly, Manipur. The stem has a woody base. The species Name *birmanicum* indicates that it was first found in Burma. It has lance-shaped leaves with serrated margins. Flower-heads appear in corymbs at the end of branches. Flowers are quite fragrant, and appear like purplish buds with white threads projecting out. Commonly known in Manipuri as *Langthrei, it is used as an offering to Gods.*

Medicinal Uses:
Leaf juice is applied to the body in burning sensations. Leaf extract with milk is a remedy for leucorrhea. The extract with honey is given in stomach ulcers.

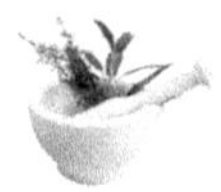

Quick Weed

Botanical Name:

Galinsoga parviflora

Family:

Asteraceae (**Sunflower family**)

Synonyms:

Tridax parviflora

Common Names:

Quick Weed, Gallant soldier, Potato weed, Small-flower galinsoga • Manipuri: *Hameng shampakpi* • Tamil: *Mookuthi Poo*

Description:

Quick Weed is a slender annual herb 20-70 cm tall, found mostly 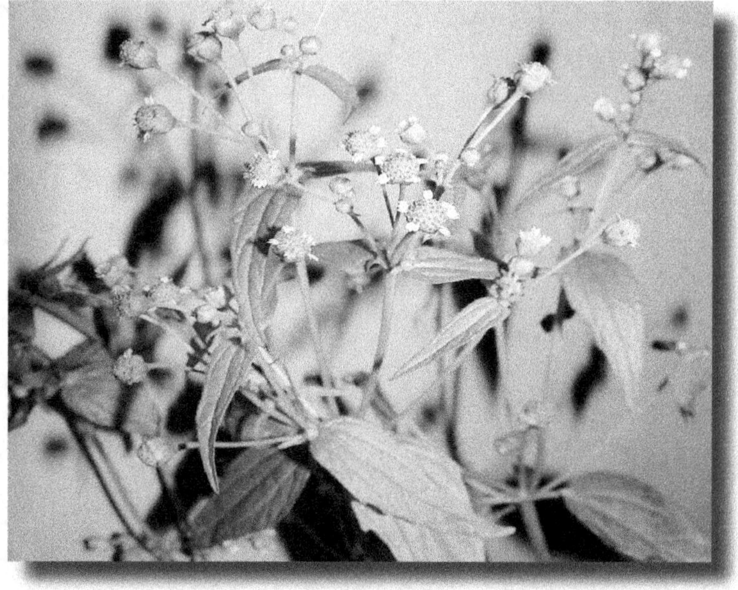 in North-east India. Leaves ovate or narrowly ovate, 2-5 cm long, 1-3 cm wide, margins serrulate or entire. Flower-heads 3-4 mm high, peduncles appressed pubescent or glandular villous; involucral bracts 2-3 mm long; ray florets white, 5 per head, rarely pink, 3-toothed, 1-2 mm long; pappus of ray florets absent or very reduced, that of disk florets consisting of blunt-tipped, fimbriate scales. Achenes sparsely appressed pubescent or glabrous.

Medicinal Uses:

In Manipur, the extract of leaves with salt is given in fever, diarrhoea and vomitting. Leaves of this plant, along with those of *Ageratum conyzoides*, *Drymaria cordata* and ginger are made into a paste and applied as a *remedy for snakebite* by the *Khasis* and *Jaintias* of *Meghalaya*.

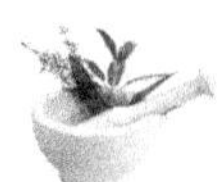

Madras Carpet

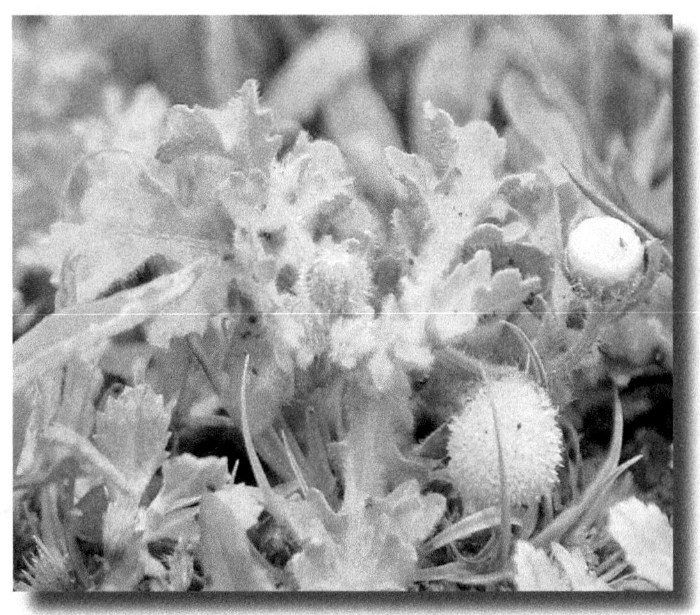

Botanical Name:
Grangea maderaspatana

Family:
Asteraceae (**Sunflower family**)

Synonyms:
Artemisia maderaspatana, Perdicium tomentosum

Common Names:
Madras Carpet • Hindi: *Mustaru, Bhediachim* • Manipuri: *Leibungou* • Marathi: *Mashipatri* • Tamil: *Masipathri* • Malayalam: *Nilampala* • Telugu: *Mastaru* • Kannada: *Davana* • Bengali: *Namuti* • Gujarati: *Jhinkimudi*

Description:
Madras Carpet is a herb commonly seen in flat bunches in harvested fields, dry river and pond beds. This hairy, branched herb spreads from the roots and grows up to 70 cm in height. The buds are white and woolly. The leaves are alternate, stalkless, deeply cut, and divided into toothed lobes. Yellow flowering heads are borne opposite the leaves, and are short- stalked, rounded, and 8-10 mm across. The flowers are small, very numerous. The involucral-bracts are ovate, thick, rigid, and hairy. The achenes are cylindric, glandular, and about 2 mm long. The papus-hairs are connate, ending in a short, fimbriate tubes.

Medicinal Uses:
Leaves are regarded in India as a *valuable stomachic* possessing *deobstruent and antispasmodic properties,* and are prescribed as an *infusion* and an *electuary* in cases of *obstructed menses* and *hysteria.*

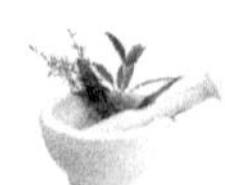

Hill Gynura

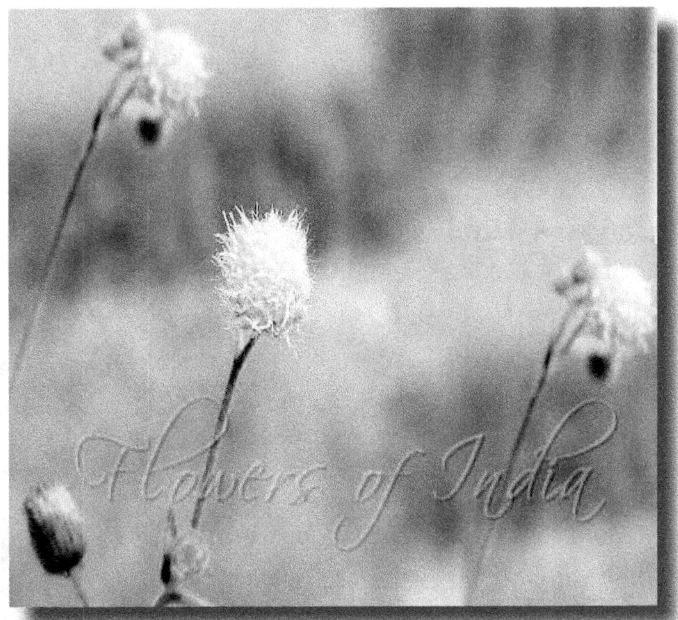

Botanical Name:

Gynura cusimbua

Family:

Asteraceae (**Sunflower family**)

Synonyms:

Gynura angulosa, Cacalia cusimbua

Common Names:

Hill Gynura • Manipuri: *Terapaibi* • Marathi: *Kusimbi*

Description:

Hill Gynura is a tall succulent herb, growing to 1-2 m tall. Angular stems are 1 cm thick, branched at the top. Alternately arranged leaves are 10-20 cm long. Upper leaves are stalkless, oblong and toothed. Lower leaves are bigger and lance-like. Numerous yellow flower-heads occur in corymsb, carried on slender peduncles. There are a few bracts below the flower-heads. Flowers are 1.5-2 cm across. This herb is commonly found in roadsides, fields and grassy slopes in Imphal and other places of Manipur. Flowering: August-November.

Medicinal Uses:

The *juice of the stem and leaves* are applied to *fresh wounds for stopping bleeding and fast healing* in traditional medicines. The *leaf paste* is also applied on the *forehead to relieve headaches* and used as *sedative drugs* by the local people.

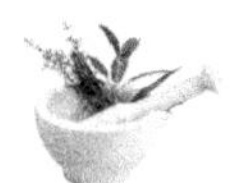

Stem Clasping Ligularia

Botanical Name:
Ligularia amplexicaulis

Family:
Asteraceae (**Sunflower family**)

Common Names:
Stem Clasping Ligularia, Ligularia

Description:
A perennial that grows to 1.0 meter high by 0.5 meters wide. The leaves are large and green, and seem to clasp the stem. Flowers are carried on erect stems above the foilage. The flowers are large, shaggy, narrow-petalled yellow daisies 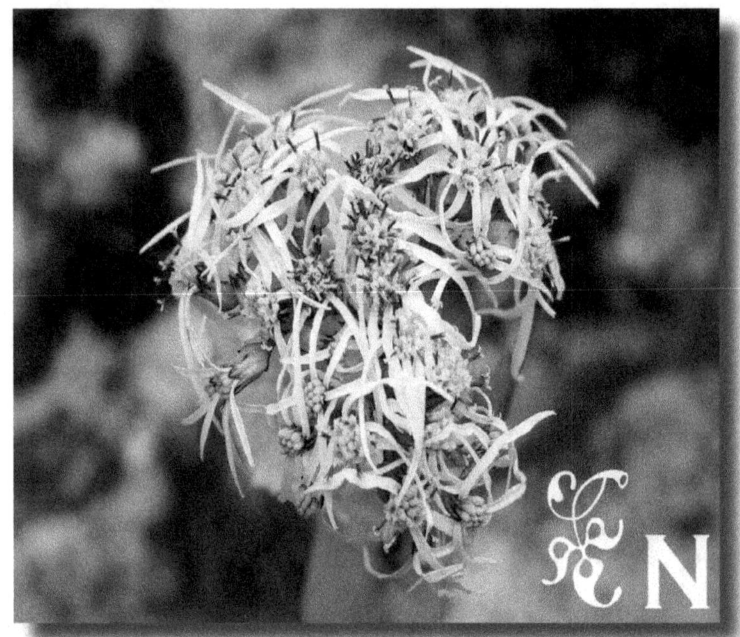 which appear in loose, flat-topped sprays in mid-summer.

Medicinal Uses:
The *stems, leaves and flowers* are used in *Tibetan medicine,* and they are said to have an *astringent taste* and a *cooling potency. Digestive* and *emetic,* they are used in the treatment of *vomiting* from *indigestion.*

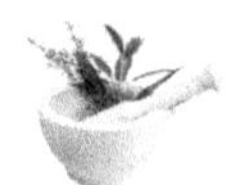

Costus

Botanical Name:

Saussurea costus

Family:

Asteraceae **(Sunflower family)**

Synonyms:

Aucklandia costus, Aplotaxis lappa, Saussurea lappa

Common Names:

Costus • Hindi: *Kuth*

Description:

Costus is a tall perennial herb, well known as a medicinal plant. Stems up to 2 m tall, or more. Lower leaves are long-stalked, pinnate, 30–40 cm long,

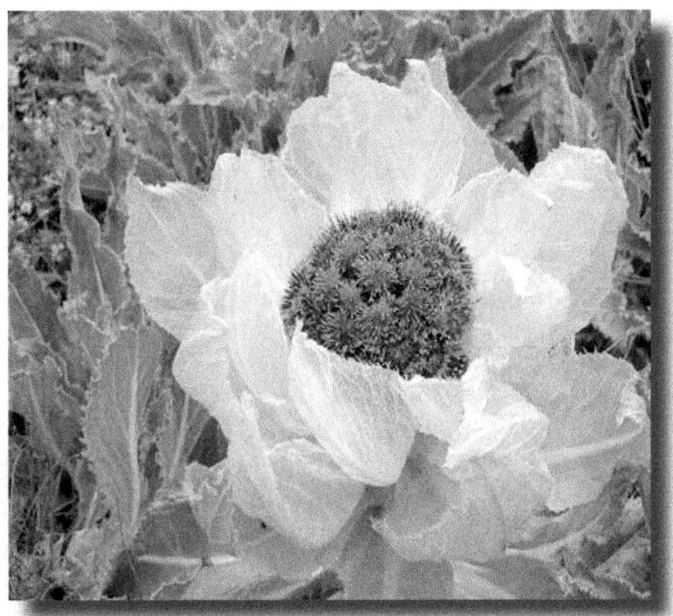

with a trianglular terminal leaflet, up to 30 cm long. Upper leaves are smaller, up to 30 cm long, stem-clasping. All leaves are irregularly toothed. There is a rounded cluster of a few purple flower-heads at the top of the stem. The flower-heads look like balls covered with purple bracts. Costus is frequently cultivated in the Himalayas as a medicinal plant. It is found in the Himalayas, from Pakistan to Himachal Pradesh, at altitudes of 2000-3300 m. Flowering: July-August.

Medicinal Uses:

Costus is widely used in several *indigenous systems of medicine* for the treatment of various ailments, like *asthma, inflammatory diseases, ulcers* and *stomach problems.*

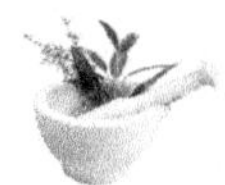

Kasturi Kamal

Botanical Name:

Saussurea gossypiphora

Family:

Asteraceae **(Sunflower family)**

Common Names:

Kasturi Kamal • Hindi: Kasturi Kamal • Nepali: Kapase phool

Description:

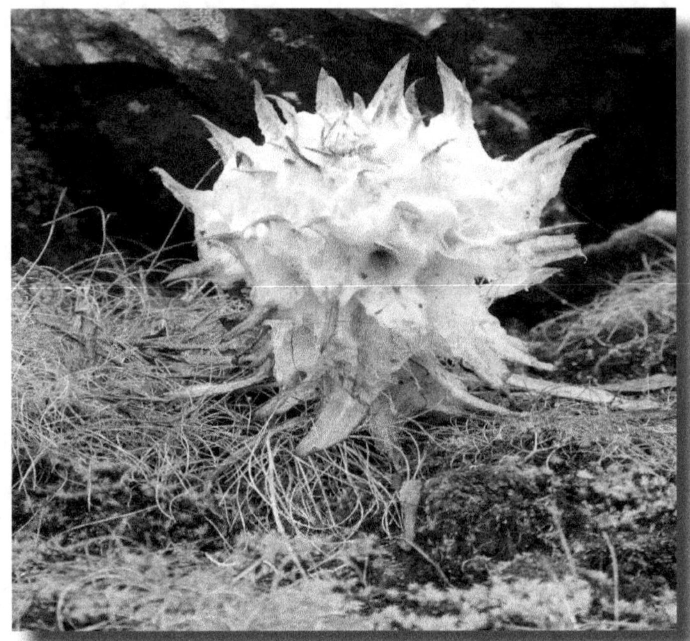

Kasturi kamal plant looks like a wooly snow-ball. It is a densely white- or grey-wooly more or less globular high altitude plant. Stem 10-20 sm, stout, hollow, enlarged club-shaped and densely leafy above, base covered with black shining leaf bases. Leaves linear, coarsely toothed or lobed, embedded in dense wooly hairs. Flower-heads purple, cylindrical 1.3-2 cm long, deeply embedded in woolly hairs and densely clustered at the top of the stem. Kasturi kamal is native to the Himalayas, and found at altitudes of 4300-5600 m.

Medicinal Uses:

The wool of this herb is applied to cuts, where it sticks compactly, seals the wound, and stops the bleeding.

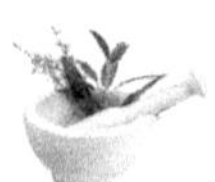

Brahma Kamal

Botanical Name:
Saussurea obvallata

Family:
Asteraceae (**Sunflower family**)

Common Names:
Hindi: Brahma Kamal

Description:
The Brahma Kamal, the much reverred flower of the Himalayas, is an excellent example of plant life at the upper limit of high mountains (3,000–4,600 m). The flowerheads are actually purple, but are enclosed in layers of greenish-yellow, papery, boat-shaped bracts.

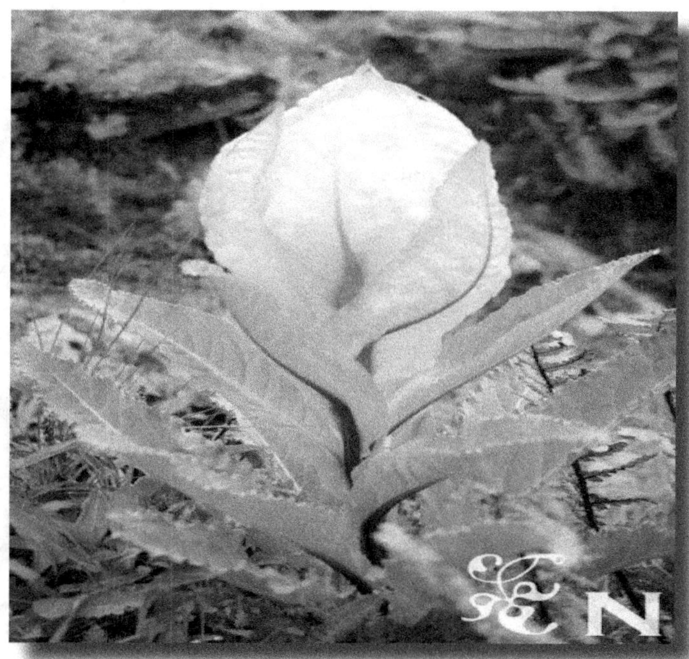

Medicinal Uses:

The flowers bloom at the height of the monsoons and are abundant in high-altitude places like *The Valley of Flowers*. The bract-cover provides the warm space needed to bloom in the cold mountains. The flowers are used as offering in the hill temples, like the shrines of *Badrinath*. The thick curved root of the plant is applied to *bruises and cuts,* as part of *local medicine.* Brahma Kamal is the *state flower of Uttarakhand.*

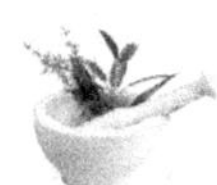

Snow Lotus

Botanical Name:

Saussurea tridactyla

Family:

Asteraceae (**Sunflower family**)

Common Names:

Snow Lotus

Description:

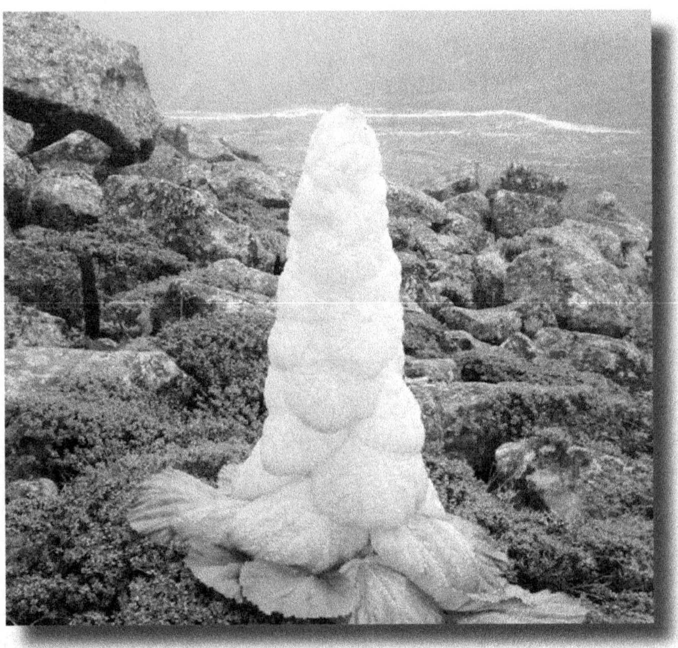

Snow Lotus was discovered by Bower at an elevation of 19,000 ft. In parts of Sikkim, where Himalayan conditions of climate prevail, we have a completely different class of flora. This where plants like the Snow lotus are found. The snow lotus is a high altitude plant (over 12,000 feet above sea level) with brilliant white flowers appearing over dark green leaves which grow through the rocks of mountain peaks. The flowers form in a dense head of small capitula, often completely surrounded in dense white to purple woolly hairs; the individual florets are also white to purple. The wool is densest in the high altitude species, and aid in thermoregulation of the flowers, minimising frost damage at night, and also preventing ultraviolet light damage from the intense high altitude sunlight. The term Snow Lotus is also used for related species S. involucrata and S. laniceps.

Medicinal Uses:

The whole plant is harvested in July and August to yield the herb that is used as a *tonic for weakness*, a *therapy for menstrual disorders*, and a *remedy for arthritis*. Due to the harsh environment of the snow lotus and the strong demand for its use in traditional herbalism, the *Snow Lotus* has *become quite rare*. It is a *native to the Himalayas*.

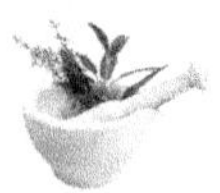

Naturopathy

St. Paul's Wort

Botanical Name:
Sigesbeckia orientalis

Family:
Asteraceae **(Sunflower family)**

Synonyms:
Siegesbeckia orientalis, Minyranthes heterophylla

Common Names:
St Paul's Wort, Indian weed • Hindi: *Lechkuri, Gobariya, Liskura, Lichakura* • Marathi: *Katampu* • Tamil: *Karuntumpai* • Nepali: *Dudhe Jhaar*

Description:
St Paul's Wort is a small annual herb, growing up to 2-4 ft tall.

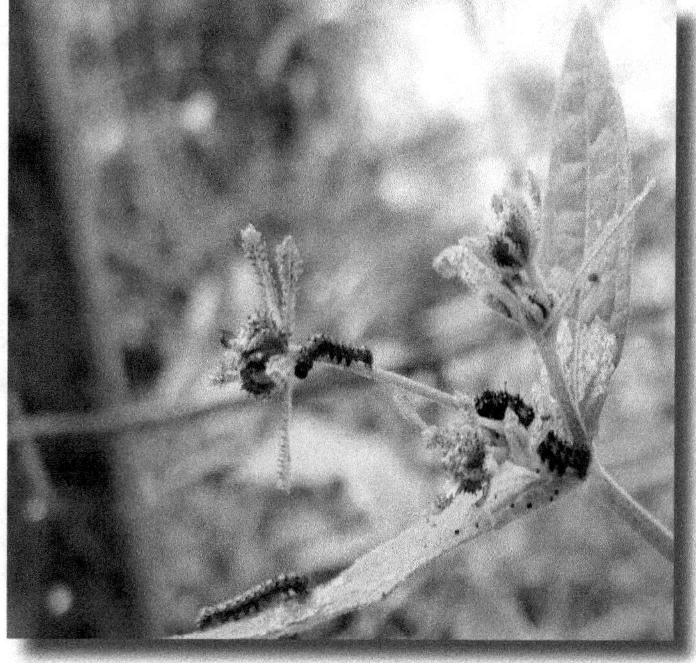

Stem and branches are velvety, purple. Oppositely arranged leaves, 5-10 cm long, are triangular-ovate, sharp tipped, with toothed margin. The flowers heads are small with five bracts just below them, which are covered with very sticky glandular hairs. The secretion continues till after the fruit is ripe and aids in its distribution - the whole flower-head breaks off and attaches itself to some passing animal. The flowering heads are yellow, small, somewhat rounded, and 5-6 mm in diameter. The ray flowers are red beneath, very short, curved back, and 3-toothed. The achenes are each enclosed in a boat-shaped bractlet which is hairless but slightly rough. St Paul's Wort is found in India at altitudes of 400-2700 m. Flowering: October-November.

Medicinal Uses:
The juice of the fresh herb is used as a *dressing for wounds*, over which, as it dries, it leaves a *varnishing coating*. A decoction of the leaves and young shoots is used as a *lotion for ulcers* and *parasitic skin diseases*.

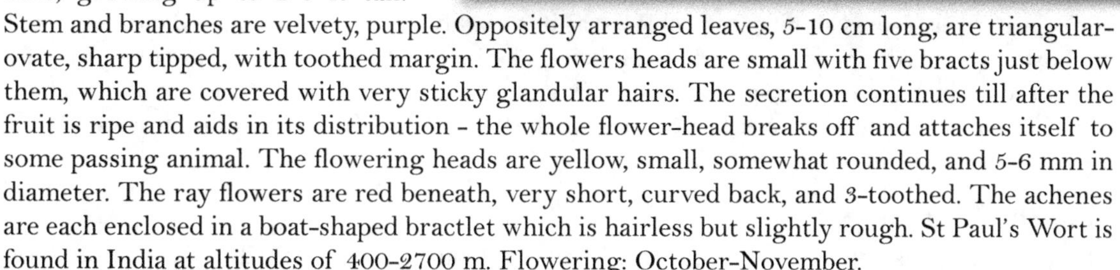

Prickly Sow-Thistle

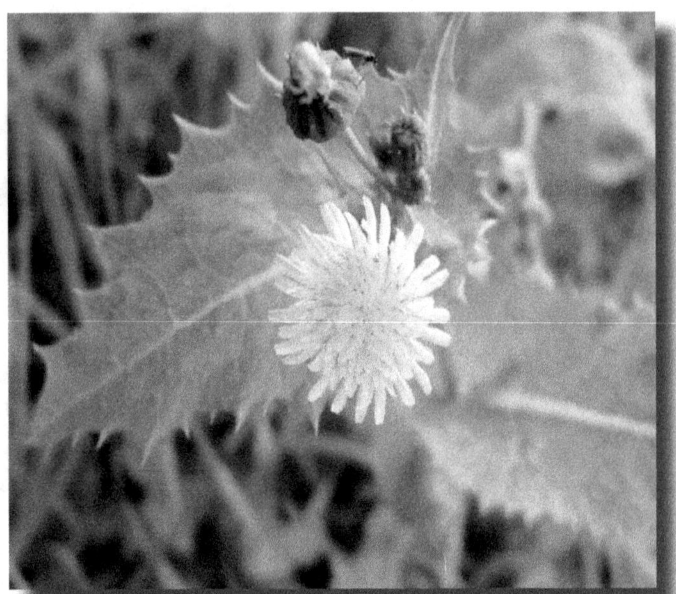

Botanical Name:

Sonchus asper

Family:

Asteraceae (**Sunflower family**)

Common Names:

Prickly Sow-Thistle, Spiny sowthistle
• Hindi: *Didhi* • Manipuri: *Khomthokpi*
• Marathi: *Mhatara*

Description:

Prickly Sow-Thistle is a creeping rooted annual, growing 1–5 ft tall. Its stems branch near the top, while its leaves, which have weak marginal prickles, clasp the stem. Plants contain a bitter milky juice. Flowers are golden-yellow, up to 1 in broad. It is a common weed throughout India and most frequently occurs on roadsides, cultivated, waste and fallow ground, field margins, meadows, ditches, and neglected areas. It often appears in pastures and crops, however it rarely causes significant problems, as it is readily grazed in pasture and out-competed by most crops. Seeds showing parachute of hairs The Prickly Sow-Thistle is spread entirely by seed. Seeds, which are, on average, 3mm long by 2 mm wide, are equipped with a small parachute of hairs, that can carry them over large distances in strong winds. Seeds lying on the ground may also be transported in moving water.

Medicinal Uses:

This *plant extract* is applied to *fresh injuries*. Plants are pounded and applied to *wounds and boils*. This herb is used as an *emollient*, i.e., a *lotion* for healing cuts, wounds and injuries.

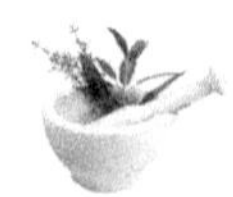

Sow Thistle

Botanical Name:

Sonchus oleraceus

Family:

Asteraceae (**Sunflower family**)

Common Names:

Hare's-lettuce, Milk thistle, Sow thistle • Hindi: *Dudhi* • Manipuri: *Khomthokpi*

Description:

The plant is an erect annual with simple branches. One particular feature about this sow thistle is that most of the plant is smooth and glabrous - without any hair or bristles. The stem is hollowed, and

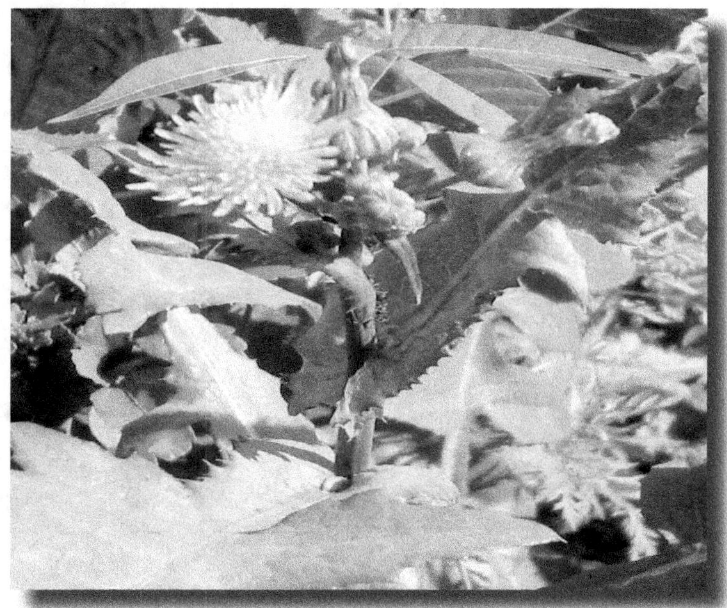

have a milky sap and its lower part usually gets a purple-brown colour later in spring. The leaves differ according age. The old (and hence lower) leaves are stalked, elongated and deeply lobed. In fact each lobe, nearly oppositely arranged along the leaf rachis, may appear to be a distinct leaf on its own. There are usually 2, 3 or 4 pairs of lobes per leaf and the terminal apical lobe is the largest and have a shape of a rounded arrow. The younger leaves also possess similar but smaller lobes. However these leaves are sessile, and have characteristic two pointed lobes (auricles) embracing the stem. Colour of the leaves vary from pale green to green-blue and may have a serrated outline but no prickles or hair. The fruits are simple achenes, brownish in colour, and oval/oblong in shape. They are wrinkled and possess obscure longitudinal ribs. At the apex they have a beakless pappus which helps seed dispersal by wind. The shape of involucral fruit is vase like - round bottomed with tapering apex and so differs from the cylindrical shape of the bud.

Medicinal Uses:

The *plant* is useful in *liver diseases*. Leaves and roots are used in *indigestion* as *febrifuge*, *stem is used as sedative, tonic*, the *root extract* is used in *ointments for ulcers and wounds*. Gum produced by *evaporating latex* is used for *ascites* and *hydrothorax*.

East Indian Globe Thistle

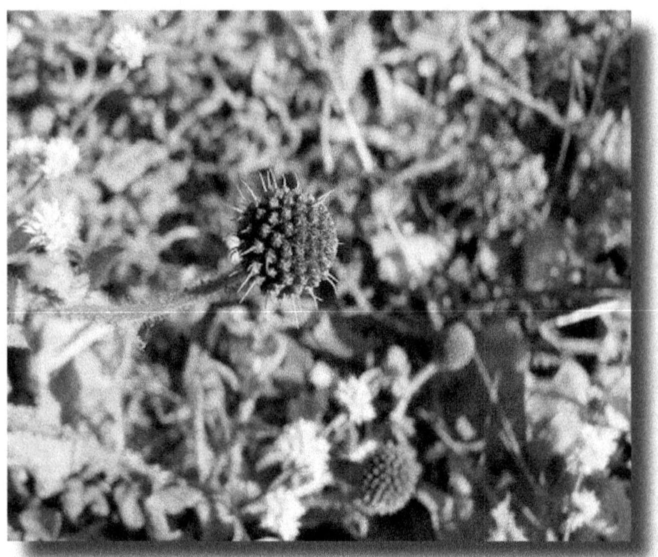

Botanical Name:
Sphaeranthus indicus

Family:
Asteraceae (**Sunflower family**)

Common Names:
East Indian Globe Thistle, Indian sphaeranthus • Hindi: *Chhagul-nudi, Gorakhmundi* • Marathi: *Gorakhmundi* • Tamil: *Visnukkarantai* • Malayalam: *Mirangani, Adakkamanian* • Telugu: *Boddatarapu* • Kannada: *Mundi* • Bengali: *Murmuriya* • Urdu: *Kamdaryus* • Gujarati: *Gorakhmundi* • Sanskrit: *Mahamundi, Tapasvini, Palankasha*

Description:
The East Indian Globe Thistle is a much branched, strongly-scented annual herb with winged stem and the wings toothed. Alternately arranged obovate-oblong leaves are narrowed at the base, dentate and serrate, 1–3 cm long. Flowers occur in purple spherical heads, 8–15 mm, consisting of numerous tiny flowers. Flowers are purple and the stamens pale-purple. Flowering: October-January.

Medicinal Uses:
According to *Ayurveda*, this herb is *hot, laxative, digestible, tonic, fattening, alterative, anthelmintic* and *alexipharmic*. It is used in *insanity, tuberculosis, indigestion, bronchitis, spleen diseases, elephantiasis, anaemia, pain in* the *uterus and vagina, piles, asthma, leucoderma, dysentery, vomiting, hemicrania,* etc.

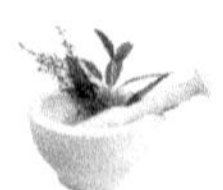

Feverfew

Botanical Name:

Tanacetum parthenium

Family:

Asteraceae (**Sunflower family**)

Synonyms:

Chrysantheim parthenium, Pyrethrum parthenium

Common Names:

Feverfew, Featherfew, Featherfoil, Febrifuge plant, Midsummer daisy, Nosebleed, Wild chamomile, Wild quinine

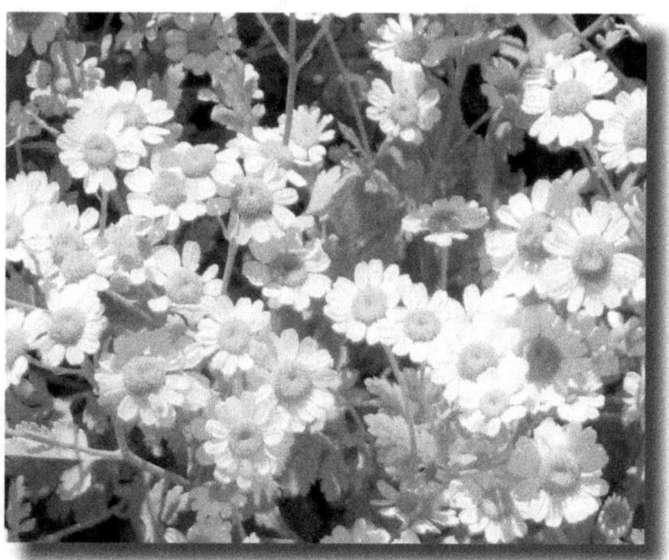

Description:

Feverfew is a traditional medicinal herb which is found in many old gardens, and is also occasionally grown for orNament, which are then used in Christmas trees. Feverfew is herbaceous and perennial plant. The plant grows into a small bush up to around 18 inches high, with citrus-scented leaves and is covered by flowers reminiscent of daisies. It spreads rapidly, and they will cover a wide area after a few years. Leaves are ovate, pinnately cut, basal, hairy and up to 3 inches long, with 3 to 5 scalloped sections. Daisy-like flowerheads with white ray and yellowish disc florets to 1 inch across are held in dense corymbs. Various cultivars have been developed for orNamental purposes.

Medicinal Uses:

Feverfew has been used for *reducing* fever, for treating *headaches*, *arthritis* and *digestive problems*. It is hypothesised that by inhibiting the release of *serotonin* and *prostaglandins*, both of which are believed to aid the onset *of migraines, feverfew* limits the *inflammation of blood vessels in the head.*

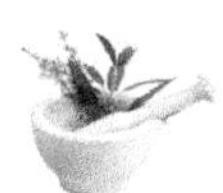

Giant Mexican Sunflower

Botanical Name:

Tithonia diversifolia

Family:

Asteraceae (**Sunflower family**)

Common Names:

Giant Mexican Sunflower, Japanese sunflower, Shrub sunflower, Tree marigold • Manipuri: Lam numitlei • Marathi: Kanak gol

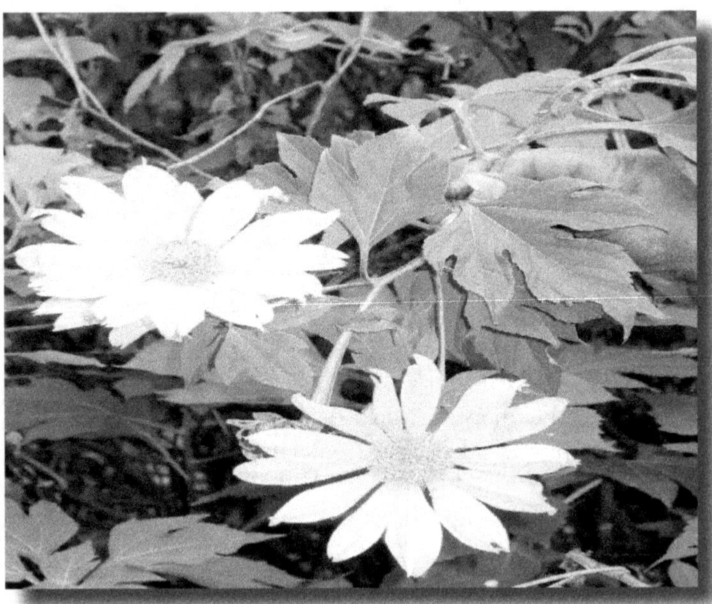

densely hairy. Alternately arranged broadly ovate leaves (lobed or simple) are 15-25 cm long. Large single flower-heads are orange-yellow, 10-15 cm across. In Manipur, flower-heads are used for wounds and bruises.

Description:

Giant Mexican Sunflower is an impressive member of the sunflower family, Asteraceae. tithonia was named for Tithonus, a legendary Trojan loved by the dawn goddess Eos, who turned him into a grasshopper. Giant Mexican sunflower is a perennial native of Mexico and Central America and is naturalized in India. It is a tall shrub, 1-3 m high. Stem is stout, erect, densely hairy. Alternately arranged broadly ovate leaves (lobed or simple) are 15-25 cm long. Large single flower-heads are orange-yellow, 10-15 cm across.

Medicinal Uses:

In Manipur, *flower-heads* are used for *wounds and bruises.*

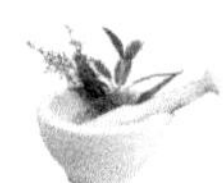

Little Ironweed

Botanical Name:
Vernonia cinerea

Family:
Asteraceae **(Sunflower family)**

Common Names:
Little ironweed, Purple fleabane • Hindi: *Sahadevi* • Marathi: *Sadodi* • Tamil: *Puvamkuruntal* • Telugu: *Sahadevi* • Bengali: *Kuksim*

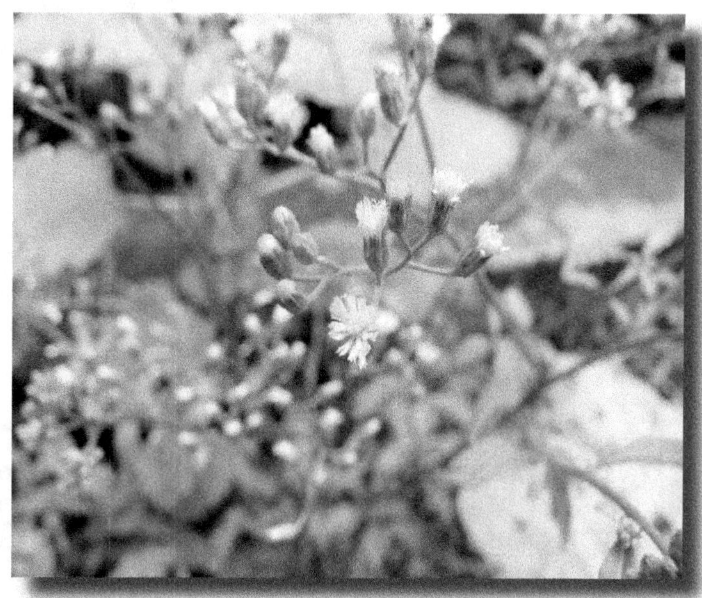

Description:
Little ironweed is an annual or short-lived perennial to 50cm with ovate leaves. The stems branch repeatedly at the top to hold aloft the small cylindrical, purple flower heads. Flowers throughout the year. Originally from Central America, now a pantropical weed, it is sometimes considered native to Western Australia. Found in upland crop areas, waste places and roadsides throughout India.

Medicinal Uses:
The *seeds* yield a *fatty oil* and are used as *an anthelmintic* and *alexipharmic.* They are said to be quite effective *against roundworms* and *threadworms.* They are also given for *coughs, flatulence, intestinal colic* and *dysuria,* and for *leucoderma, psoriasis* and other *chronic skin diseases. The seeds are made into a paste with lime juice* and used for *destroying pedicles.*

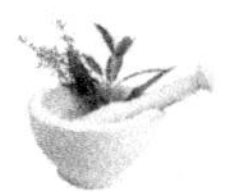

Chinese Wedelia

Botanical Name:
Wedelia chinensis

Family:
Asteraceae (**Sunflower family**)

Synonyms:
Solidago chinensis

Common Names:
Chinese Wedelia • Hindi: *Pilabhangara, Bhanra* • Marathi: *Pivala-Bhangra* • Tamil: *Manjalkarilamkanni, Patalai kayyantakarai* • Malayalam: *Mannakkannunni* • Telugu: *Guntagalagara* • Kannada: *Gargari, Kalsarji* • Bengali: *Bhimra* • Konkani: *Birimgarsi* • Sanskrit: *Pitabhrnga, Pitabhrngarajah*

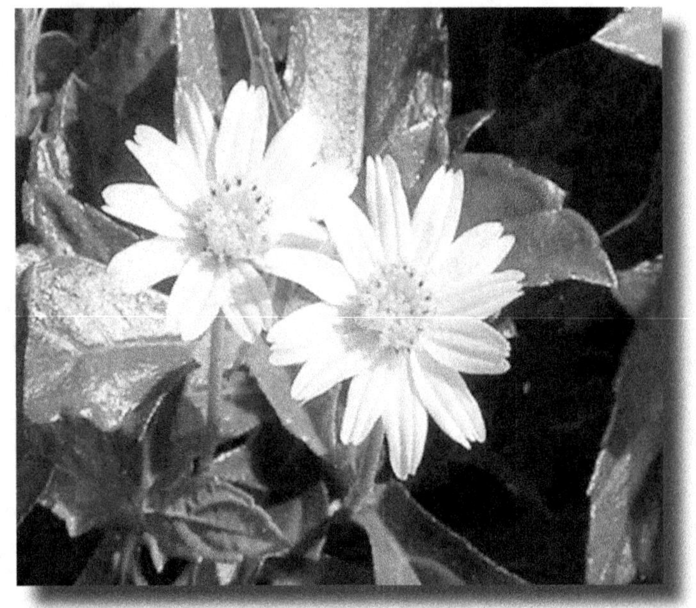

Description:
Chinese Wedelia is a tender, spreading, and hairy herb, with the branches usually less than 50 cm long. The leaves are oblong to oblong-lanceolate, 2-4.5 cm in length, and narrowed at both ends. The margins are entire or obscurely toothed; and both surfaces are covered with sharp-pointed, appressed, straight, and stiff hairs. The heads are stalked, about 1 cm in diameter, and yellow. The involucral bracts are oblong-ovate. The ray flowers are 8-12, spreading, about equal to the bracts, and broad; the disk flowers number about 20, and are short, narrow, and pointed. The achenes are nearly cylindric, and hairy.

Medicinal Uses:
The leaves are used in *dyeing grey hair* and in *promoting the growth of hair*. They are considered *tonic, alternative*, and useful in *coughs, cephalalgia, skin diseases*, and *alopecia*. The juice of the leaves is much used as a *snuff in cephalalgia*. The seeds and flowers, as well as the leaves, are used in decoction, in the quantity of half of teacupful twice daily, as a deobstruent. *In decoction, the plant is* used *in uterine haemorrhage and menorrhagia.*

Yellow Dots

Botanical Name:

Wedelia trilobata

Family:

Asteraceae (**Daisy/Sunflower family**)

Common Names:

Yellow Dots, Creeping daisy, Wedelia

Description:

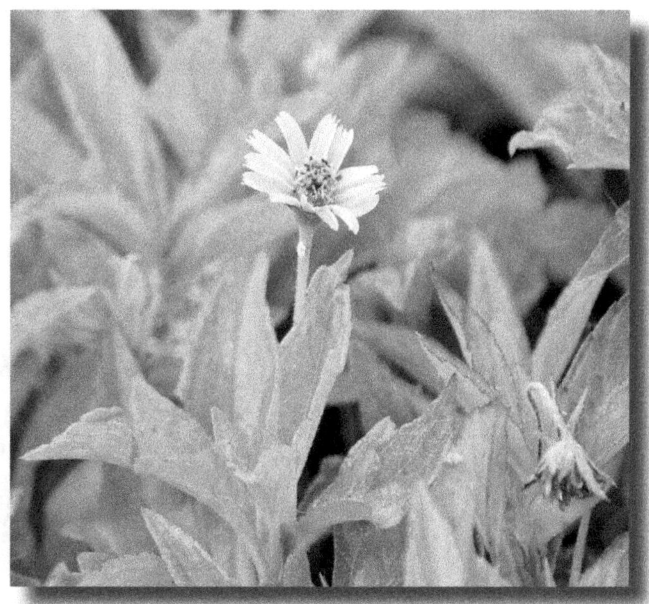

Yellow Dots is native to the northern part of South America and the West Indies. It is a creeping evergreen perennial that roots at the leaf nodes and spreads widely. The leaves are ovate and usually 3 lobed. The flower is a yellow daisy-like flower that is approximately 1 inch across. Plant creeps and roots at nodes, making a dense ground cover, as well as a great hanging basket. It grows well under trees but it will not tolerate wet soils.

Medicinal Uses:

In traditional medicine, Wedelia is used to treat *hepatitis, liver and stomach infections* and to clear the *placenta after birth.*

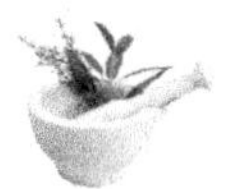

"

East Himalayan Balsam

Botanical Name:

Impatiens arguta

Family:

Balsaminaceae (**Balsam family**)

Synonyms:

Impatiens gagei

Common Names:

East Himalayan Balsam

Description:

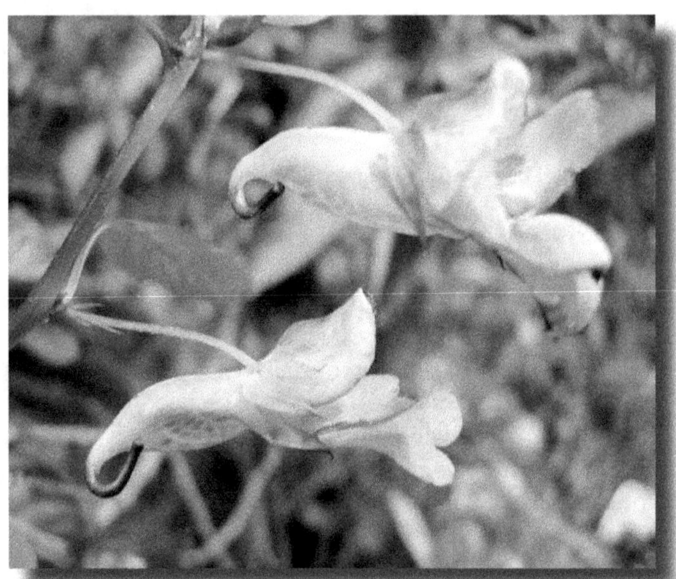

East Himalayan Balsam is a beautiful wildflower found in the forests, thickets, grasslands in valleys, along canals and moist places, in East Himalayas, from E. Nepal to NE India, at altitudes of 1800-3200 m. It is a perennial plant, growing up to 70 cm tall. Erect stems are rigid and branched. Alternately arranged leaves, carried on 1-4 cm long stalks, are ovate or ovate-elliptic, 4-15 cm long, and 2-4.5 cm broad. Leaf margins are sharply toothed, and the tip is pointed or tapering. Flowers arise singly or doubly in leaf axils. Flower stalks are long, slender, often with 2 bracts at base. Flowers are pink or purple-red, large or medium- sized. Flowers are characterized by lower lobes of the lateral petals being divided into two. Lateral sepals are 4 - outer 2, with tip long cuspidate - inner 2, narrowly lanceshaped. Lower sepal is sac-like, narrowed into an incurved, short spur. Upper petal is circular. Lateral united petals are not clawed, 2-lobed. Basal lobes are broadly oblong; Farther lobes are shaped like the head of an axe, large, with a two parted tip. Flowering: July-October.

Medicinal Uses:

The flowers are used medicinally for *dissolving clots, promoting diuresis,* and *treating abdominal pain, postpartum blood stasis, carbuncles,* and *difficulty in urination.*

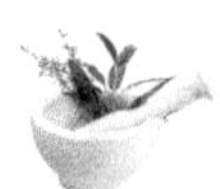

Chitra

Botanical Name:

Berberis aristata/chitria

Family:

Berberidaceae (**Barberry family**)

Common Names:

Chitra, Indian barberry, Tree turmeric, Nepal barberry • Hindi: *Chitra* • Tamil: *Mullukala* • Malayalam: *Maramanjal* • Bengali: *Darhaldi*

Description:

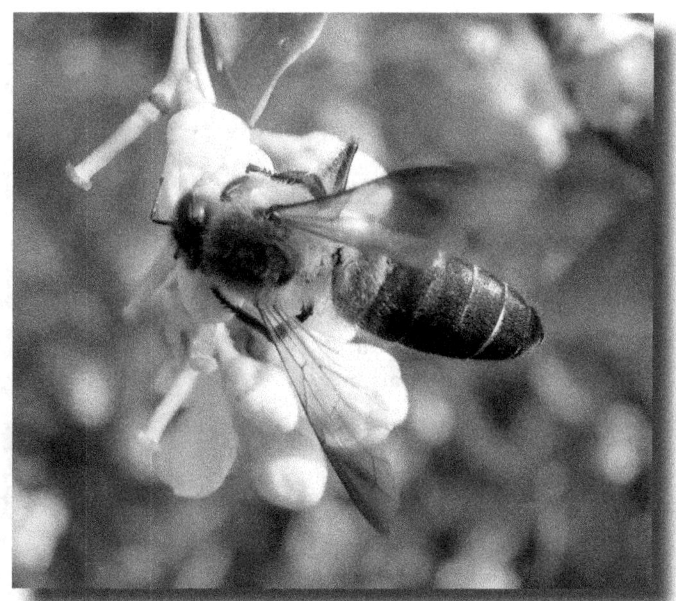

Chitra is an evergreen shrub found commonly in Garhwal and Himalayas. It grows to 4 m high and 0.5 m wide. Leaves, in tufts of 5-8, lance-like, simple spiny, toothed, leathery, stalkless, pointed, 4.9 cm long, 1.8 cm broad, deep green on the dorsal surface and light green on the ventral surface. Spines (which, in fact, are modified leaves) are three-branched and 1.5 cm long. Flowers, stalked, yellow, in simple to corymbose raceme, with 11-16 flowers per cluster. The average diameter of a fully opened flower is 12.5 mm. Six yellow sepals (3 small, 3 large), with 6 petals, yellow, 4-5 mm long.

Medicinal Uses:

It is one of very important medicinal plants. Almost every part of this plant has some medicinal value. A bitter tonic antiperiodic and diaphoretic An infusion is used in the treatment of *malaria, eye complaints, skin diseases, menorrhagia, diarrhoea* and *jaundice*. Berberine, universally present in rhizomes of Berberis species, has marked *antibacterial effects*. Since it is not appreciably absorbed by the body, it is used orally in the treatment of various *enteric infections*, especially *bacterial dysentery*.

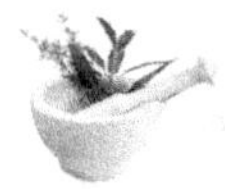

Indian Barberry

Botanical Name:

Berberis lycium

Family:

Berberidaceae (**Barberry family**)

Common Names:

Indian Barberry, Boxthorn Barberry • Hindi: *Darhaldi, Chatrol* • Kumaon: *Kirmora* • Urdu: *Ishkeen, Kushmul, Zarch* • Gujarati: *Kasmal*

Description:

Indian Barberry is a semi deciduous shrub, 2–4 m high, leaves lanceolate or narrowly obovate-oblong, entire or with a few large spinous teeth, arranged alternately on stem. Inflorescence a raceme, flowers 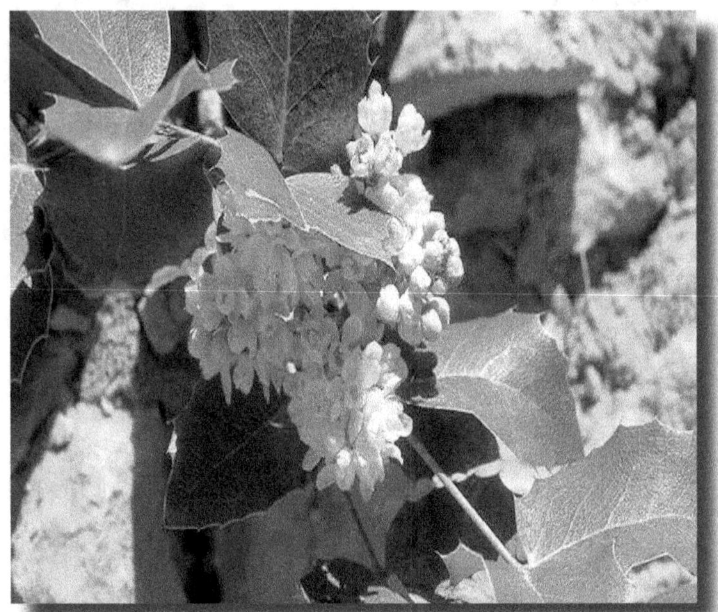 yellow born in axillary clusters longer than the leaves. Fruit, berries, black. Flowering: March–June.

Medicinal Uses:

The Indian Barberry's roots are used as a remedy for *swollen and sore eyes, broken bones, wounds, gonorrhoea, curative piles, unhealthy ulcers, acute conjunctivitis* and in *chronic ophthalmia*. It is also used as a *bitter tonic astringent, diaphoretic* and *febrifuge*. The leaves are given in *jaundice*.

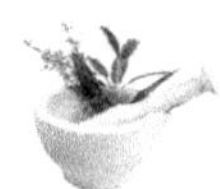

Nepal Mahonia

Botanical Name:
Mahonia napaulensis

Family:
Berberidaceae (**Barberry family**)

Common Names:
Nepal Mahonia, Indian Barberry

Description:
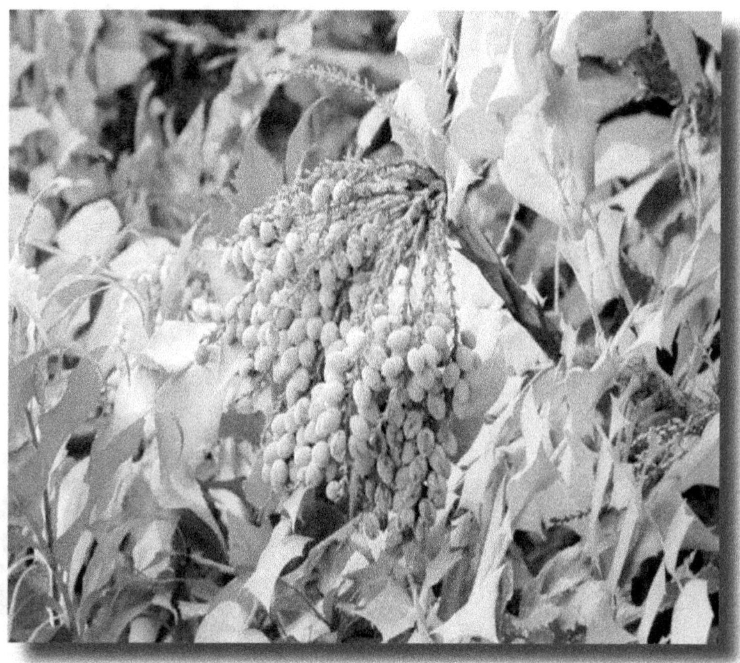

Indian barberry is an evergreen shrub growing to 2.5m by 3m, with large, pinnately compound leaves. The leaves are about 18 in (46 cm) long with 9 to 13 stiff, sharply spiny, hollylike leaflets. The fragrant lemon-yellow flowers, appearing in late winter, are borne in erect racemes 3-6 in (7.6-15 cm) long. The fruit is a berry, first green, then turning bluish black with a grayish bloom. They are about a half inch long and hang in grapelike clusters. It is in leaf all year, in flower from March to April. Fruit is eaten raw or cooked. An acid flavour, but it is rather nice raw especially when added to muesli or porridge. Unfortunately, there is relatively little flesh and a lot of seeds. The fruit can also be dried and used as raisins.

Medicinal Uses:

The fruits are said to be *diuretic* and *demulcent*. They are used in the *treatment of dysentery. Berberine, universally present in rhizomes of the Mahonia species,* has marked *antibacterial effects* and is used as a *bitter tonic.*

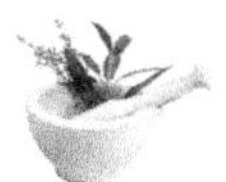

Calabash Tree

Botanical Name:
Crescentia cujete

Family:
Bignoniaceae (**Bignonia family**)

Common Names:
Calabash tree • Tamil: *Tiruvottukkay* • Kannada: *Sokeburude*

Description:
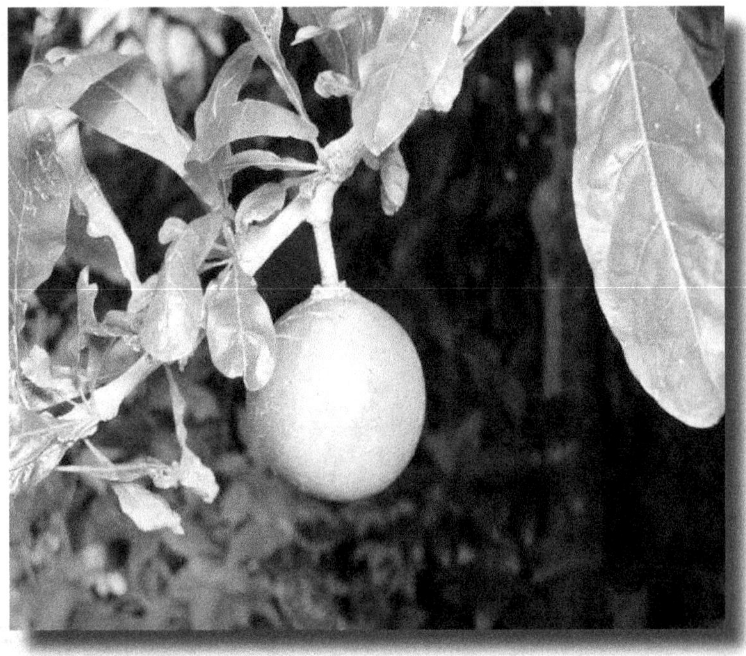

The Calabash tree is a small tree of multiple uses, originating from tropical America, now widely distributed in the tropics. The calabash tree grows to 30 feet often with multiple trunks. The rangy twisting branches have simple elliptical leaves clustered at the nodes. The greenish-yellow flowers are marked with purple veins. The flowers arise from the trunk or main branches and appear from May through January. The woody fruit, botanically a capsule, is elliptic, ovate, or spherical and may grow to 10 inches in diameter. The fruit takes up to seven months to ripen. Fibers from the calabash tree were twisted into twine and ropes. The hard wood made tools and tool handles. The split wood was woven for sturdy baskets. But it was the calabash's gourd-like fruit that made the plant truly useful. Large calabashes were used as bowls and, peculiarly, to disguise the heads of hunters.

Medicinal Uses:
In the field of traditional medicine, the *fruit pulp* is used for *respiratory problems*, such as *asthma*.

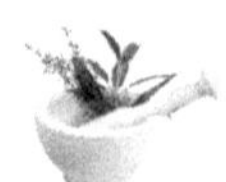

Katsagon

Botanical Name:

Fernandoa adenophylla

Family:

Bignoniaceae (**Jacaranda family**)

Synonyms:

Haplophragma adenophyllum

Common Names:

Katsagon • Hindi: *Marodphali*

Description:

This tree is fairly common in Delhi. It is 15-20 m tall, trunk 15-25 cm in diameter, large leaves 25-50 cm; leaflets 3-6 on each side of midrib, long elliptic, 8-14 X 2.5-6 cm. Large, pale yellow, trumpet

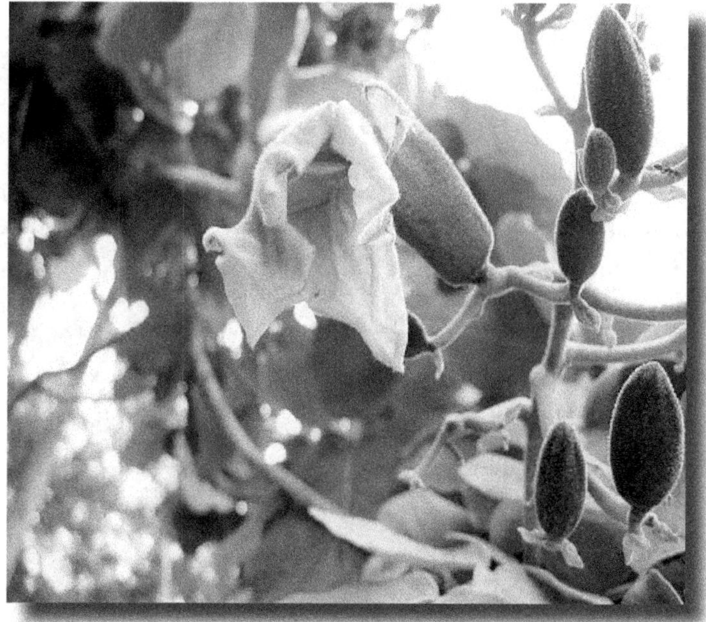

shaped flowers occur in panicles. The flowers look very similar to those of Sausage tree, except for the colour. The flowers mostly remain closed in the day and open up at night. The fruit is long and twisted, hanging like snakes from the branches.

Medicinal Uses:

The tree is extensively used in the field of *traditional medicine*. As an ingredient in massage oils, it is supposed to ease *muscular tensions*.

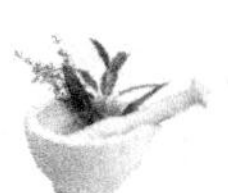

Sausage Tree

Botanical Name:

Kigelia africana

Family:

Bignoniaceae (**Jacaranda family**)

Synonyms:

Crescentia pinnata, Kigelia pinnata

Common Names:

Sausage Tree, Common Sausage Tree • Hindi: *Balam khira, Jhar fanoos* • Kannada: *Aanethoradu Kaayi, Mara Sowthae* • Telugu: *Enuga thondamu, Kijili, Naagamalle*

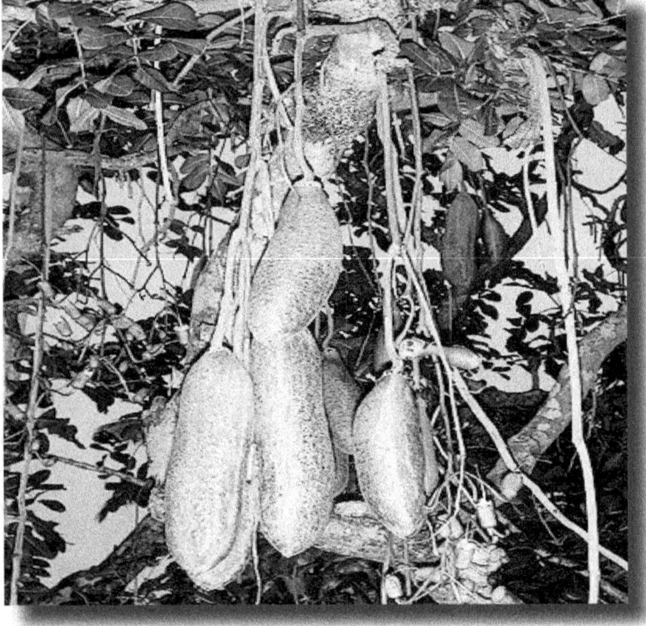

Description:

The blood-red flowers of the sausage tree bloom at night on long, ropelike stalks that hang down from the limbs of this tropical tree. The fragrant, nectar-rich blossoms are pollinated by bats, insects and sunbirds in their native habitat. The mature fruits dangle from the long stalks like giant sausages. They may be up to two feet long and weigh up to 6.8 kg. The flowers are seen hanging from the tree while they haven't opened. After they open, they fall off quite soon. The fruit, while not palatable for humans, is popular with hippos, baboons, and giraffes. Mainly grown as a curiosity and orNamental, both for its beautiful deep red flowers and its strange fruit.

Medicinal Uses:

There are also a range of traditional uses of the fruit, varying from *topical treatments for skin afflictions,* to *treatment for intestinal worms.* There are *some steroid chemicals* found in the *sausage tree* that are currently added to *commercially available shampoos* and *facial creams.*

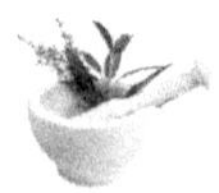

Roheda

Botanical Name:

Tecomella undulata

Family:

Bignoniaceae (**Jacaranda family**)

Synonyms:

Tecoma undulata, Bignonia undulate

Common Names:

Roheda, Honey Tree, Desert Teak, Marwar Teak • Hindi: *Roheda, Rohida* • Marathi: *Rakhtroda, Raktarohida* • Sanskrit: *Chalachhada, Dadimacchada, Dadimapuspaka*

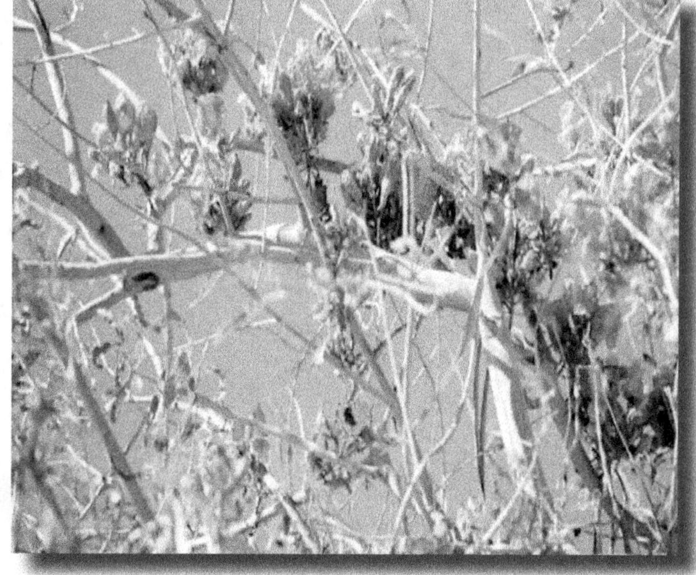

Description:

Roheda is a deciduous or nearly evergreen tree of desert or dry regions. It occurs on flat and undulating areas including gentle hill slopes and sometimes also in ravines. It thrives very well on stabilized sand dunes, which experience extreme low and high temperatures. Leaves are narrow, somewhat lance-shaped, with wavy margins, 5-12 cm long. In spring time it produces beautiful showy tubular flowers in yellow, orange and red colours. Fruit is a long, thin, slightly curved capsule up to 20 cm long, with winged seeds. Roheda is mainly used as a source of timber. Its wood is strong, tough and durable. It takes a fine finish. The wood is excellent for firewood and charcoal. Cattle and goats eat leaves of the tree. Camels, goats and sheep consume flowers and pods. Roheda plays an important role in ecology. It acts as a soil-binding tree by spreading a network of lateral roots on the top surface of the soil. It acts as a windbreak and helps in stabilizing shifting sand dunes. It is considered as the home of birds and provides shelter for other desert wildlife. Shade of tree crown is shelter for the cattle, goats and sheep during summer days.

Medicinal Uses:

The *bark obtained from the stem is used as a remedy for syphilis.* It is also used in *curing urinary disorders, enlargement of* the *spleen, gonorrhoea, leucoderma* and *other liver diseases.* The seeds are used against *abscess.*

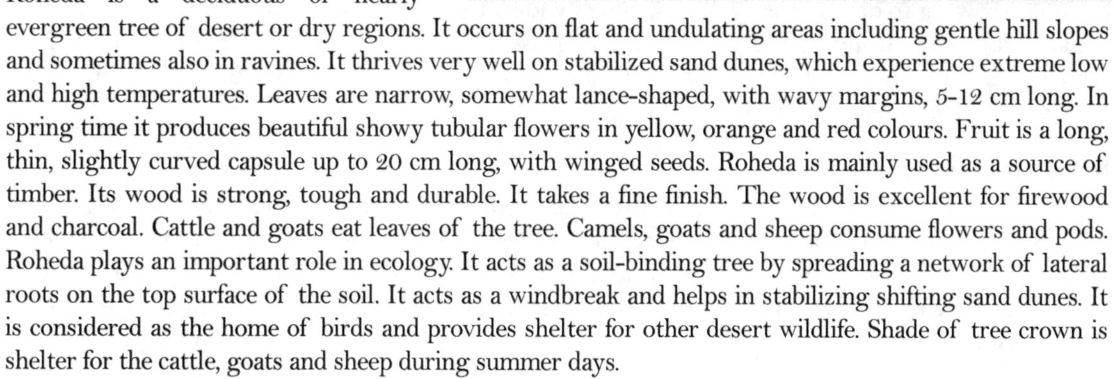

Comfrey

Botanical Name:
Symphytum officinale

Family:
Boraginaceae (**Forget-me-not family**)

Synonyms:
Symphytum uliginosum

Common Names:
Comfrey, Black root, Boneset, Common comfrey, Consolida, Consound, Knitbone, Slippery root

Description:
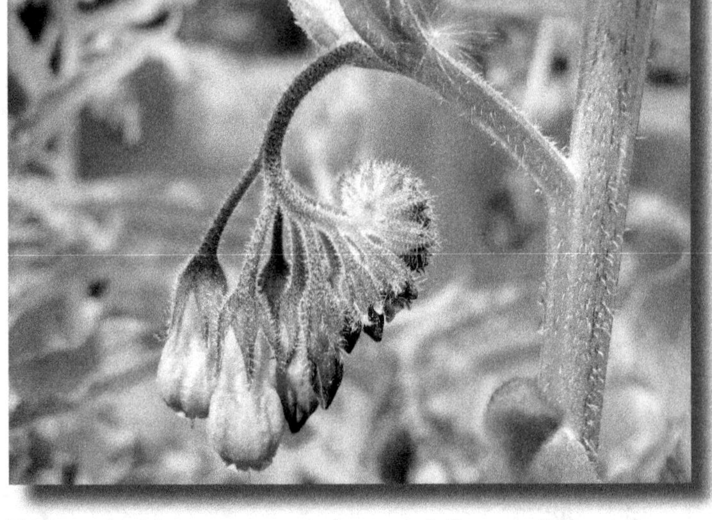

Comfrey is a perennial herb with a black, turnip-like root and large, hairy broad leaves that bears small bell-shaped white, cream, purple or pink flowers. It is native to Europe, growing in damp, grassy places, and is widespread throughout the British Isles on river banks and ditches. Comfrey has long been recognised by both organic gardeners and herbalists for its great usefulness and versatility; of particular interest is the "Bocking 14" cultivar of Russian Comfrey (Symphytum xuplandicum).

Medicinal Uses:
The *herb contains allantoin, a cell proliferant that speeds up the natural replacement of body cells.* Comfrey was used to treat a wide variety of ailments ranging from *bronchial problems, broken bones, sprains, arthritis, gastric and varicose ulcers, severe burns, acne* and other *skin conditions*. It was reputed to have bone and teeth building properties in children, and have value in treating 'many female disorders'.

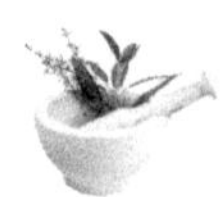

Indian Borage

Botanical Name:

Trichodesma indicum

Family:

Boraginaceae (**Forget-me-not family**)

Common Names:

Indian Borage • Hindi: *Chhota Kalpa* • Gujarati: *Undhanphuli* • Kannada: *Katte tume soppu* • Tamil: *Kallutaitumapi* • Telugu: *Guvvagutti* • Marathi: *Chota Kalpa* • Sanskrit: *Adhapuspi*

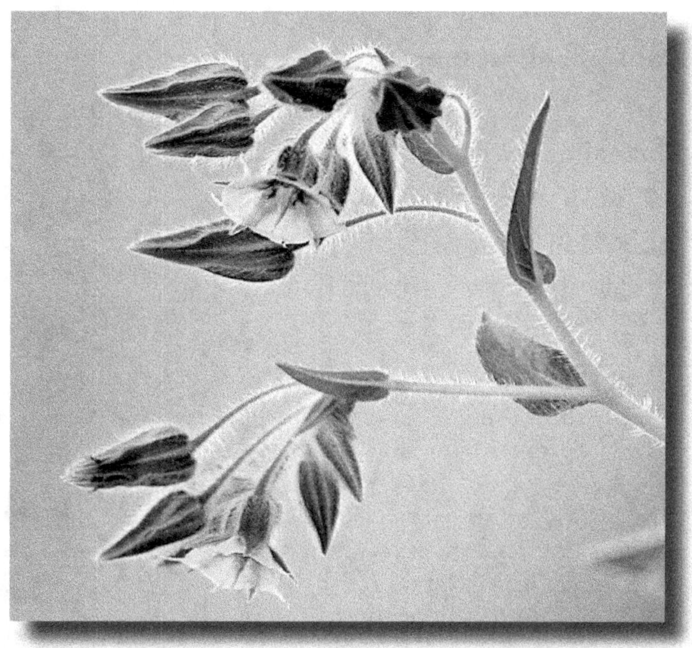

Description:

This is an erect, spreading, branched, annual herb, about 50 centimeters in height, with hairs springing from tubercles. The leaves are stalkless, opposite, lanceolate, 2 to 8 centimeters long, pointed at the tip, and heart-shaped at the base. The flowers occur singly in the axils of the leaves. The sepal tube (calyx) is green, hairy, and 1 to 13 centimeters long, with pointed lobes. The flower tube is pale blue, with the limb about 1.5 centimeters in diameter, and the petals pointed. The fruit is ellipsoid, and is enclosed by the calyx. The nutlets are about 5 millimeters long, and rough on the inner surface. It is found throughout India, on roadsides and stony dry wastelands, upto 1,500 m.

Medicinal Uses:

The plant is *acrid, bitter in taste.* In herbal medicines, it is *thermogenic, emollient, alexeteric, anodyne, anti-inflammatory, carminative, constipating, diuretic, depurative, ophthalmic, febrifuge* and *pectoral.* This herb is also used in *arthralgia, inflammations, dyspepsia, diarrhoea, dysentery, strangury, skin diseases and dysmenorrhoea.*

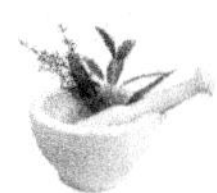

Shepherd's Purse

Botanical Name:
Capsella bursa-pastoris

Family:
Brassicaceae (**Cauliflower family**)

Common Names:
Shepherd's Purse, Cocowort, Blind weed

Description:
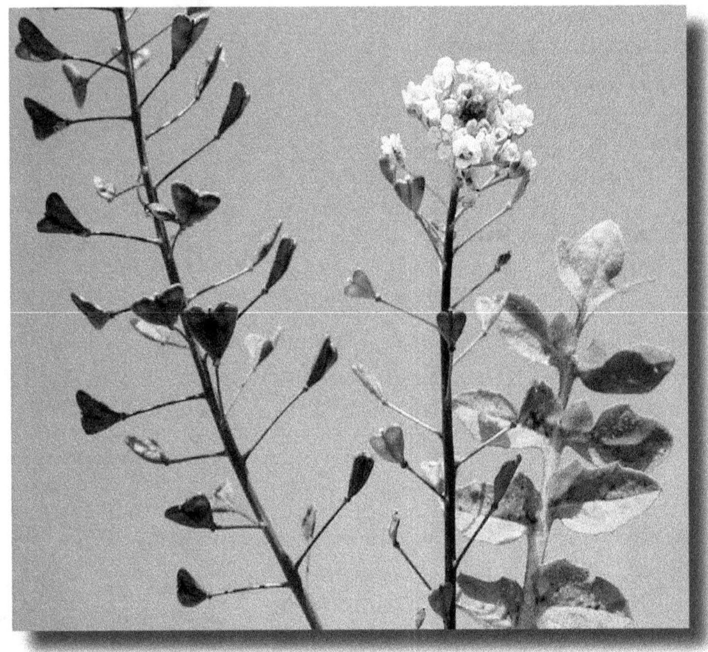

Shepherd's Purse is originally from Europe, but has become very common in many parts of the world. The species Name *bursa-pastoris* mean purse of the shepherd. This Name refers to the fruit-capsule in the shape of a triangle, attached to slender stalk from its pointy end, with a notch on the top. Shepherd's Purse grows in gardens, fields, waste grounds, and embankments with soils that are not too dry and that provide enough sunshine. This is rather a small plant, growing to 6-20 cm high. The basal leaves are lanceolate and dentate. The white flowers are arranged in loose racemes. Flowers are radially symmetrical with four petals. The seeds of this plant give off a viscous compound when moistened. Aquatic insects stick to it and eventually die. This can be used as a mosquito control method, killing off the mosquito larvae, and makes it a borderline carnivorous plant. The seeds, leaves, and root of this plant are edible. *In China, it is commercially grown for consumption.* Flowering: December-January.

Medicinal Uses:
In Manipur, it is being used to stop *bleeding from internal organs.*

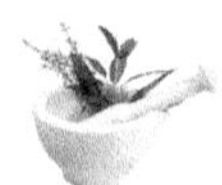

Indian Olibanum

Botanical Name:

Boswellia serrata

Family:

Burseraceae **(Torchwood family)**

Common Names:

Indian Olibanum, Indian frankincense •Hindi: *Kundur, Luban, Salai* • Kannada: *Dupa, Guggala, Guggaladupa, Kunda, Lobana* •Malayalam:*Kunturukkam, Mukundam, Palankam, Parankisamprani* • Marathi: *Salaphali, Saalayi* • Sanskrit: *Agavrttika, Ashvamutri, Asraphala, Bahusrava, Gajabhaksha* • Tamil: *Attam, Kunduru, Kundurukkan, Kungiliyam* •Telugu: *Anduga, Dhupamu, Guggilamu, Parangisambrani*•Urdu: *Kundur, Lobana*

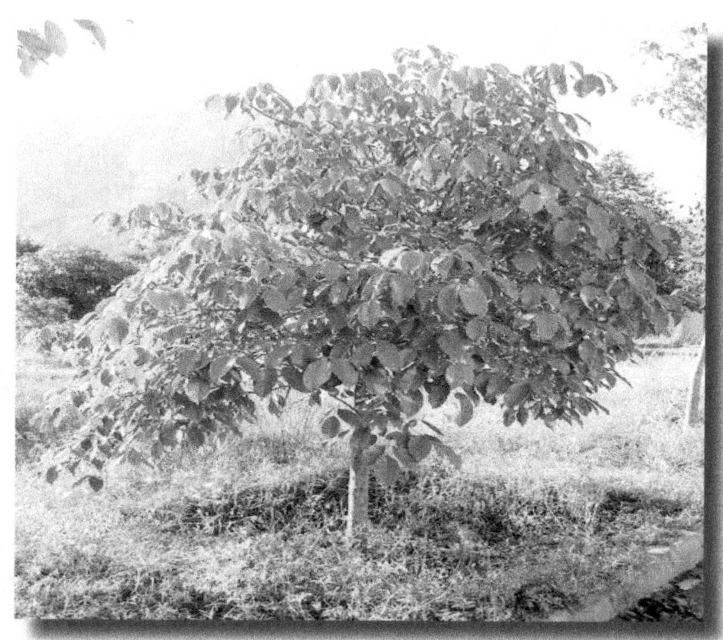

Description:

Indian Olibanum is a deciduous tree endemic to India and has been recorded on dry hills and slopes, on gravelly soils between an altitude range of 275-900 m. It is a medium sized tree, 3-5 m tall, with ash coloured papery bark. Alternately arranged leaves are pinnate, crowded at the end of branches, 20-40 cm long. There are 8-15 pairs of leaflets, 3-6 cm long, with an odd one at the tip. Leaflets are ovate, with toothed margin. Flowers are tiny, creamy, about 8 mm across, borne in 10-15 cm long racemes in leaf axils. There are 10 stamens with a short style and a 3-lobed stigma. Fruits are 2 cm long, 3-cornered. Indian Olibanum tree, on injury, exudates an oleo-gum-resin known as Salai, Guggal or Indian Frankincense. Flowering: January.

Medicinal Uses:

Extracts of Indian Olibanum have been clinically studied for *osteoarthritis and joint function*, particularly for *osteoarthritis of the knee*. A Boswellia extract marketed under the name, *Wokvel* has undergone *human efficacy, comparative, pharmacokinetic studies*. The Indian Olibanum is used in the manufacture of the supposed *anti-wrinkle agent, 'Boswelox'*, which has been criticised as being ineffective.

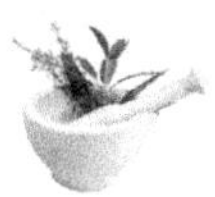

Hatchet Cactus

Botanical Name:

Pelecyphora aselliformis

Family:

Cactaceae (**Cactus family**)

Synonyms:

Mammillaria aselliformis, Anhalonium aselliforme, Ariocarpus aselliformis

Common Names:

Hatchet Cactus, Peyotillo, Woodlouse cactus

Description:

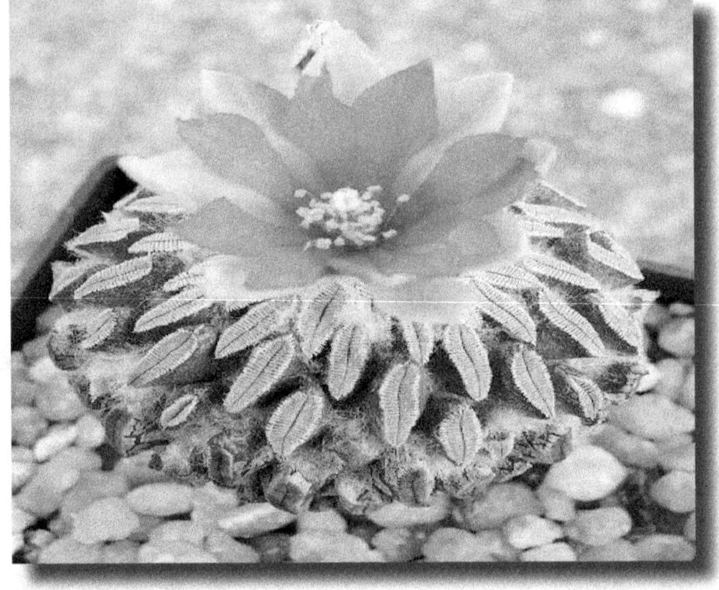

Native to Mexico, Hatchet Cactus is a cylindric cactus with flattened elongated tubercles, arranged in spirals, and 40-60 spines. It presents a heavy and fleshy root and grayish green stem, globular when young but becoming cylindrical soon, of about 10 cm high and between 5 and 6 cm. wide. The areolas are woolly at first and present a great amount of small, non sharp spines, joined together with the base with the tip free. The flowers appear on apex, between the wool of the young areolas. They measure about 3 cm. wide and are violet. It is a very rare plant, since it grows very slowly and send offsets after many years only. Flowering: February-October.

Medicinal Uses:

Hatchet Cactus is a well known medicinal peyote sold in the markets of San Luís Potosí, Mexico, and is used as a remedy for *fevers* and *rheumatic pains*. Extracts have also been shown to have *antibiotic activity*.

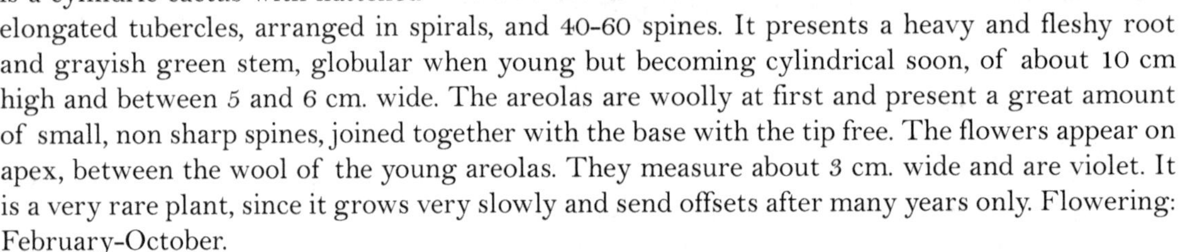

Fever Nut

Botanical Name:

Caesalpinia bonduc

Family:

Caesalpiniaceae (**Gulmohar family**)

Synonyms:

Caesalpinia crista, Caesalpinia bonducella, Guilandina bonduc

Common Names:

Yellow Nicker, Gray nicker, Nicker seed, Bonduc nut, Fever nut, Nicker bean • Hindi: *Kantkarej, Kantikaranja, Kuberakshi* • Marathi: *Sagarlata* • Tamil: *Kalichchikkai* • Malayalam: *Kalanchi* • Telugu: *Gachchakaya* • Kannada: *Gajikekayi* • Sanskrit: *Latakaranjah, Kuberakshi, Kantakikaranjah*

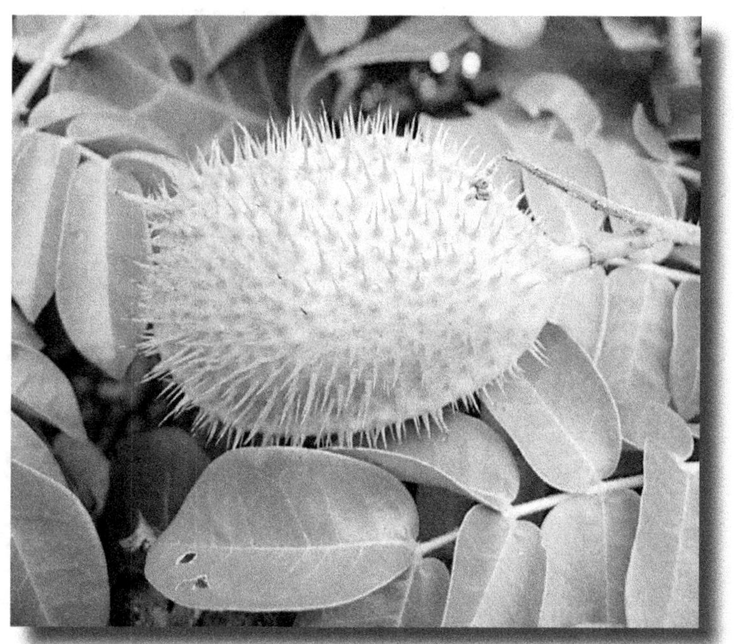

Description:

Yellow Nicker is a large, thorny, straggling, shrub which behaves like a strong woody climber, taking support of trees. The branches are armed with hooks and straight hard yellow prickles. Leaves are large, double compound, with 7 pairs of pinnae, and each with 3-8 pairs of leaflets with 1-2 small recurved prickles between them on the underside. Flowers are yellow, in dense long-stalked racemes at the top. Fruits are inflated pods, covered with wiry prickles. Seeds are 1-2 per pod, oblong or globular, hard, grey with a smooth shiny surface. The hard and shiny seeds are green, turning grey. They are used for jewellery.

Medicinal Uses:

Fruits are *tonic and antipyretic. Seeds yield a fatty oil* used as a *cosmetic* and for *discharges* from the ear. Leaves and bark are febrifuge.

Amaltas

Botanical Name:

Cassia fistula

Family:

Caesalpiniaceae (**Gulmohar family**)

Common Names:

Amaltas, Golden shower tree, Indian Laburnum • Hindi: *Amaltas* • Manipuri: *Chahui* • Tamil: *Konrai* • Malayalam: *Vishu konnai* • Marathi: *Bahava* • Mizo: *Ngaingaw* • Bengali: *Sonali, Bandarlati, Amultas* • Urdu: *Amaltas*

Description:

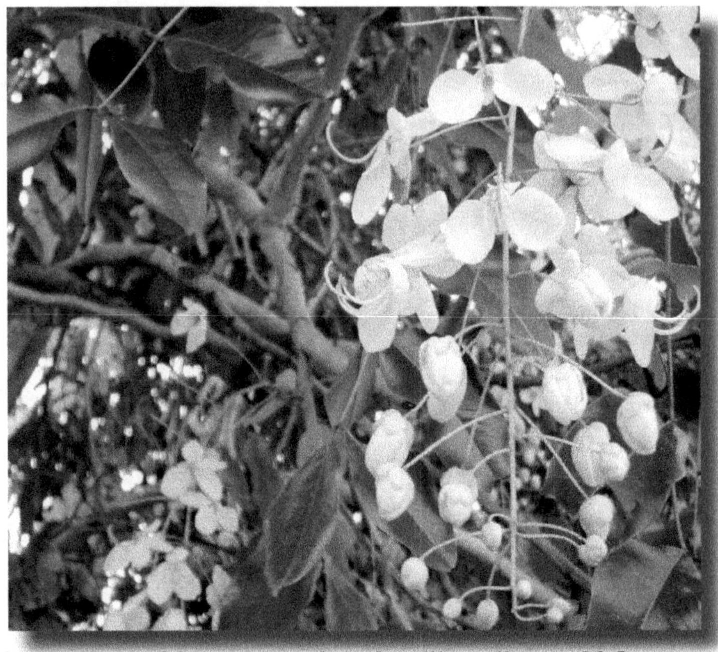

This native of India, commonly known as *Amaltaas*, is one of the most beautiful of all tropical trees when it sheds its leaves and bursts into a mass of long, grape-bunches like yellow gold flowers. A tropical orNamental tree with a truck consisting of hard reddish wood, growing up to 40 feet tall. The wood is hard and heavy; it is used for cabinet, inlay work, etc. It has showy racemes, up to 2" long, with bright, yellow, fragrant flowers. These flowers are attractive to bees and butterflies. The fruits are dark-brown cylindrical pods, also 2' long, which also hold the flattish, brown seeds (up to 100 in one pod) These seeds are in cells, each containing a single seed.

Medicinal Uses:

The *sweet blackish pulp of the seedpod* is used as a *mild laxative.*

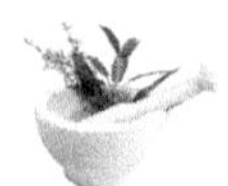

Coffee Senna

Botanical Name:

Cassia occidentalis

Family:

Caesalpiniaceae (**Gulmohar family**)

Synonyms:

Senna occidentalis

Common Names:

Coffee Senna, Coffeeweed, Negro coffee • Hindi: *Kasunda, Bari kasondi* • Marathi: *Ran-takda, Kasivda, Kasoda, Rankasvinda* • Tamil: *Nattam takarai, Payaverai* • Malayalam: *Mattantakara* • Telugu: *Thangedu* • Kannada: *Kolthogache* • Bengali: *Kalkashunda* • Oriya: *Kasundri* • Urdu: *Kasonji* • Assamese: *Hant-thenga* • Gujarati: *Kasundri* • Sanskrit: *Kasamarda, Vimarda, Arimarda*

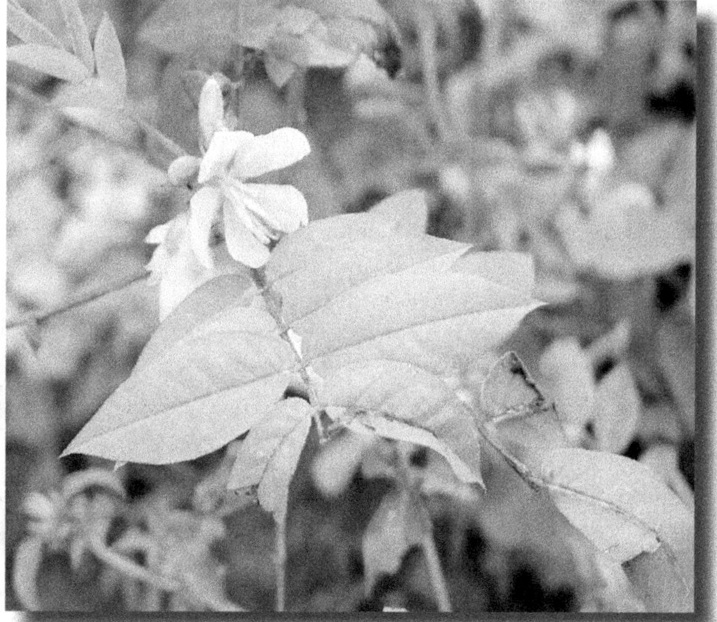

Description:

Coffee Senna is a smooth annual that can grow up to 2 m tall. The leaves are compound, leaflets, in 4-6 pairs, have a sharp tip. These leaflets are 2-9 cm long and 2-3 cm wide with a distinct gland 3-5 mm from the base of the stalk. Flowers occur in leaf axils. Sepals are green and 6-9 mm long. The petals are yellow and 1-2 cm long. The 6-7 stamens are of two different lengths. The seed pods are dark brown, 8 to 12 cm long, 7-10 mm wide and curve slightly upward. The seeds are dull brown, 4-5 mm long and flattened on both ends. The seeds can be roasted and made into a coffee-like drink.

Medicinal Uses:

The seed is bitter and has purgative properties. It is also used as a diuretic, liver detoxifier, as a hepato-tonic (balances and strengthens the liver). Further, used in whooping cough and convulsion.

Sita Ashok

Botanical Name:

Saraca indica/Jonesia asoka

Family:

Caesalpiniaceae (**Gulmohar family**)

Common Names:

Sita Ashok, Sorrowless tree • Hindi: Sita Ashok, Ashok • Gujarati: Ashopalava • Kannada: Achenge • Malayalam: Hemapushpam • Marathi: Jasundi • Tamil: Asogam • Telugu: Asokamu

Description:

Ashoka is one of the most legendary and sacred trees of India, and one of the most fascinating flowers in

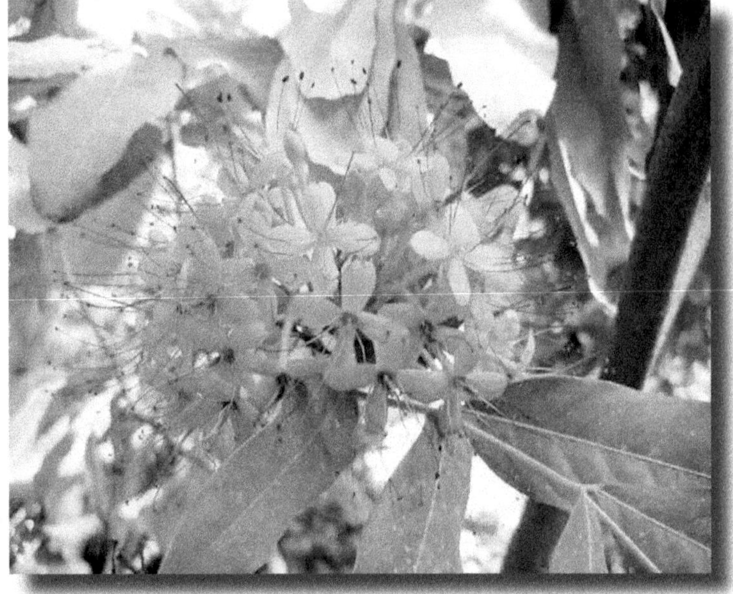

the Indian range of flower essences. Ashok is a Sanskrit word meaning without grief or that which gives no grief. Indigenous to India, Burma and Malaya, it is an erect tree, small and evergreen, with a smooth, grey-brown bark. The crown is compact and shapely. Flowers are usually to be seen throughout the year, but it is in January and February that the profusion of orange and scarlet clusters turns the tree into an object of startling beauty. Pinned closely on to every branch and twig, these clusters consist of numerous, small, long-tubed flowers which open out into four oval lobes. Yellow when young, they become orange then crimson with age and from the effect of the sun's rays. From a ring at the top of each tube spread several long, half-white, half-crimson, stamens which give an hairy appearance to the flower clusters. In strong contrast to these fiery blooms is the deep-green, shiny foliage. The foot-long leaves each have four, five or six pairs of long, wavy-edged, leaflets. Young leaves are soft, red and limp and remain pendent even after attaining full size.

Medicinal Uses:

As one would expect from a tree of the country it has many useful medicinal properties. The juice obtained from *boiling the bark* is a cure for *some ailments of women,* and *a pulp of the blossoms* is one of the remedies used for *dysentery.*

Tanner's Cassia

Botanical Name:

Senna/Cassia auriculata

Family:

Caesalpiniaceae (**Gulmohar family**)

Common Names:

Tanner's Cassia • Hindi: *Tarwar* • Marathi: *Tarwad* • Kannada: *Tangedi* • Telugu: *Tagedu* • Tamil: *Avaram* • Gujarati: *Awala* • Malayalam: *Avaram*

Description:

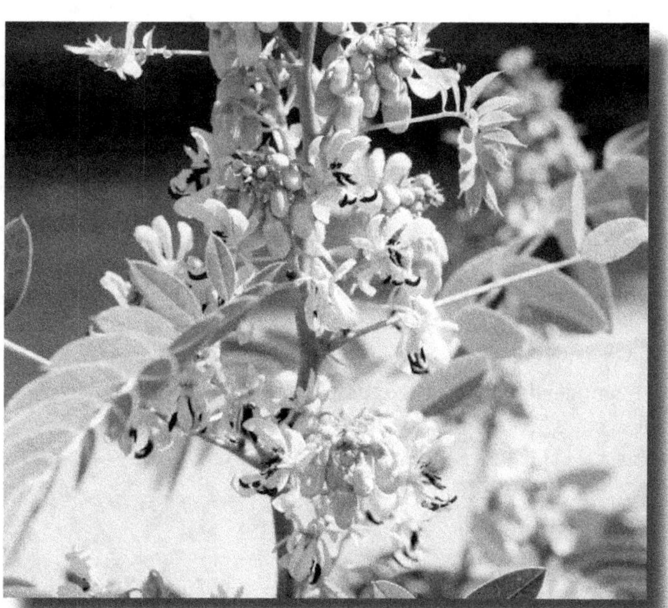

Tanner's Cassia is a branched shrub, growing upto 1-1.5 m high. It has a smooth reddish brown bark. It has many ascending branches and 8-10 cm long pinnate leaves. There are 8-12 pairs of leaflets, each 2-3 cm long. Bright yellow flowers appear in recemes at the end of branches. The flowers are 4-5 cm across. Upper three stamens are reduced to stamenoides. Fruit is a 7-12 cm long, flat brown pod.

Medicinal Uses:

In Ayurveda, the root of this plant is used in a decoction for fevers, diabetes, diseases of the urinary system and *constipation. The leaves have laxative properties.* The dried flower and flowers buds are used as substitutes.

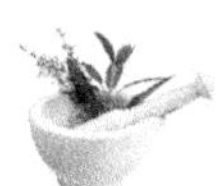

Asian Spider Flower

Botanical Name:

Cleome viscosa

Family:

Capparaceae (**Caper family**)

Synonyms:

Polanisia viscose

Common Names:

Asian spider flower, Yellow spider flower, Cleome, Tickweed • Hindi: *Bagra* • Urdu: *Hulhul* • Malayalam: *Naivela* • Tamil: *Naikkaduku* • Kannada: *Nayibela* • Gujarati: *Pilitalvani* • Telugu: *Kukkavaminta* • Marathi: *Pivala tilavan*

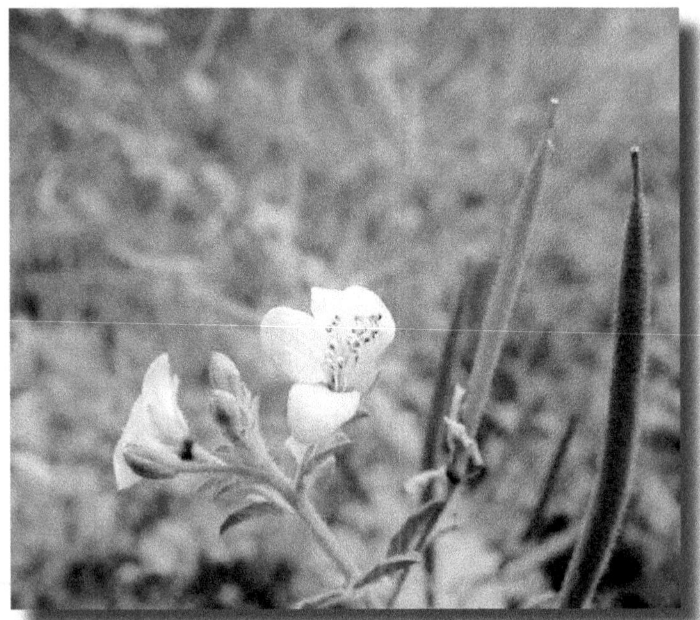

Description:

Asian spider flower is a usually tall annual herb, up to a meter high, more or less hairy with glandular and eglandular hairs. Leaves 3-5-foliolate, petiolate; leaflets obovate, elliptic-oblong, very variable in size, often 2-4 cm long, 1.5-2.5 cm broad, middle one largest; petiole up to 5 cm long. Racemes elongated, up to 30 cm long, with corym¬bose flowers at the top and elongated mature fruits below, bracteate. Flowers 10-15 mm across, whitish or yellowish; pedicels 6-20 mm long; bracts foliaceous. Sepals oblong-lanceolate, 3-4 mm long, 1-2 mm wide, glandular-pubescent. Petals 8-15 mm long, 2-4 mm broad, oblong-obovate. Stamens 10-12 (rarely more, up to 20), not exceeding the petals; gynophore absent. Fruit 30-75 mm long, 3-5 mm broad, linear-oblong, erect, obliquely striated, tapering at both ends, glandular-pubescent, slender; style 2-5 mm long; seeds many, 1-1.4 mm in diam., glabrous with longitudinal striations and transverse ridges, dark brown.

Medicinal Uses:

The leaves are *diaphoretic*, *rubefacient* and *vesicant*. They are used as an external application to *wounds* and *ulcers*. The *juice of the leaves* has been used to relieve *earaches*. The *seeds* are *anthelmintic, carminative, rubefacient* and *vesicant*. The seed contains 0.1% of *viscosic acid* and 0.04% of *viscosin*.

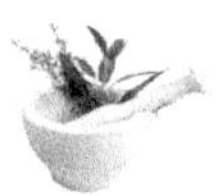

Garlic Pear Tree

Botanical Name:

Crataeva adansonii subsp. odora

Family:

Capparaceae (**Caper family**)

Common Names:

Garlic pear tree, Caper tree, Three-leaf caper, Obtuse Leaf Crateva • Hindi: *Barna, Barni* • Manipuri: *Loiyumba lei* • Tamil: *Marvilinga* • Bengali: *Barun* • Sanskrit: *Varuna* • Malayalam: *Nir mathalam* • Kannada: *Nirvala* • Telugu: *Voolemara*

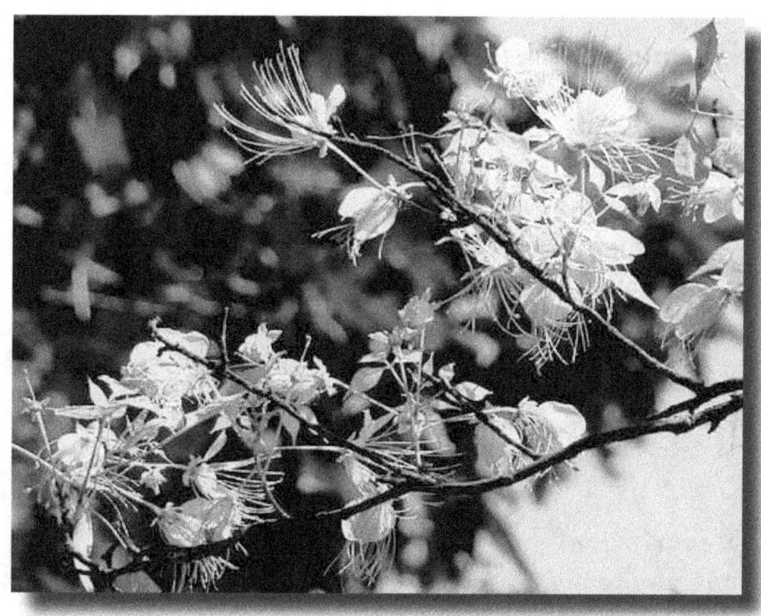

Description:

A moderate sized deciduous tree found throughout India, especially along the river banks. Bark grey, smooth horizontally wrinkled. Leaves trifoliate. Flowers white, or cream in many flowered terminal corymbs. The bark is grey, and the wood is yellowish-white, turning light-brown when old. The leaves are clustered at the ends of branchlets, with a common petiole 5 to 10 centimeters long, at the summit of which are tree leaflets. The leaflets are ovate-lanceolate or ovate, 7.5 to 12 centimeters long, 4 to 6 centimeters wide, and pointed at the base, with a rather slender point at the tip. The flowers occur in terminal corymbs, are about 5 centimeters in diameter, greenish-yellow, and the stamens are purplish. The petals are ovate or oblong, with the claw half as long as limb. The fruit is ovoid or rounded, and 3 to 5 centimeters in diameters, with hard and rough rind. The seeds are about 10 centimeters in length, numerous, kidney-shaped, and embedded in a yellow pulp.

Medicinal Uses:

It is used in Indian *Ayurvedic medicine*. It has *anti-inflammatory, diuretic, lithontriptic, demulcent* and *tonic* properties. The bark yields ceryl alcohol, friedelin, lupeol, betulinic acid and diosgenin. It is useful in disorders of *urinary organs, urinary tract infections, pains* and *burning sensations, renal* and *vesical calculi.*

Nag Kesar

Botanical Name:

Mesua ferrea

Family:

Clusiaceae **(Garcinia family)**

Common Names:

Cobra saffron, Ceylon ironwood, Indian rose chestnut • Hindi: *Nag champa, Nagkesar* • Urdu: *Narmishka* • Tamil: *Tadinangu* • Marathi: *Thorlachampa* • Malayalam: *Vainavu* • Assamese: *Nokte* • Manipuri: *Nageshor*

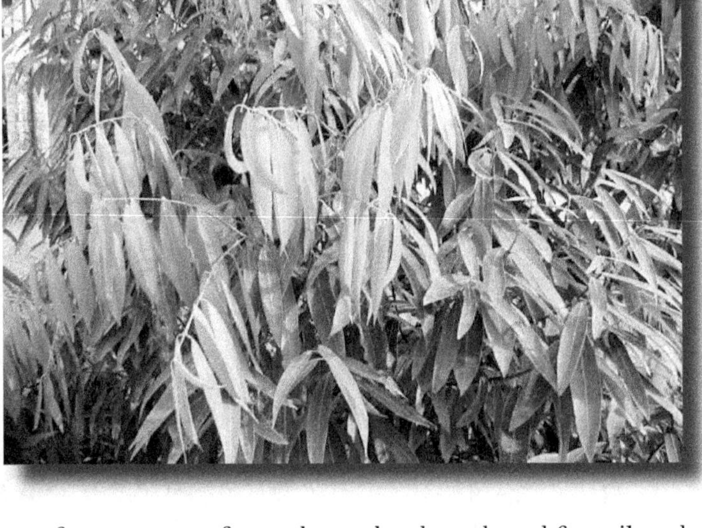

Description:

A handsome Indian evergreen tree often planted as an orNamental for its fragrant white flowers that yield a perfume; source of very heavy hardwood used for railroad ties. In olden time, the very hard timber was used for making lances. It is a small to medium-sized evergreen tree up to 13 m tall, often buttressed at the base with a trunk up to 90 cm in diameter. It has simple, narrow, oblong, dark green leaves 7-15 cm long, with a whitish underside; the emerging young leaves are red to yellowish pink and drooping. The flowers are 4-7.5 cm diameter, with four white petals and a center of numerous yellow stamens. The flowers have many uses - they are used to make an incense and also used to stuff pillows in some countries. It is the National tree of Sri Lanka.

Medicinal Uses:

The leaves are applied to the head in the form of *a poultice for severe colds*. Oil from the seeds is used for *sores, scabies, wounds* and *rheumatism*. The root of this herb is often used as an *antidote for snake poison. The dried flowers* are used for *bleeding haemorrhoids* and *dysentery with mucus*. Fresh flowers are also prescribed for *excessive thirst, perspiration, cough* and *indigestion*.

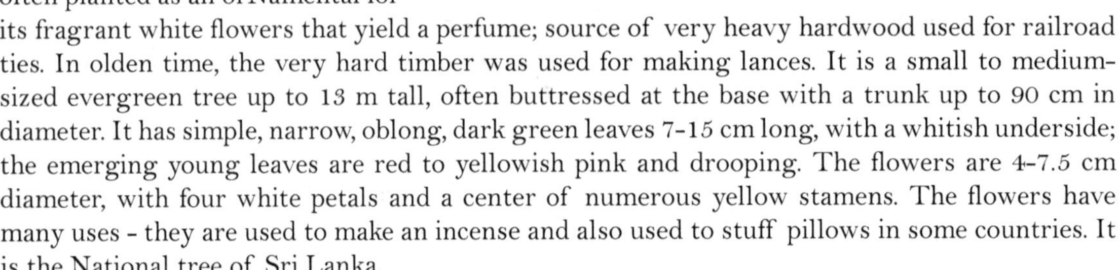

Arjun Tree

Botanical Name:

Terminalia arjuna

Family:

Combretaceae (**Rangoon creeper family**)

Common Names:

Arjun • Hindi: Arjun • Manipuri: Maiyokpha • Tamil: Marutu • Malayalam: Nirmarutu • Kannada: Nirmatti

Description:

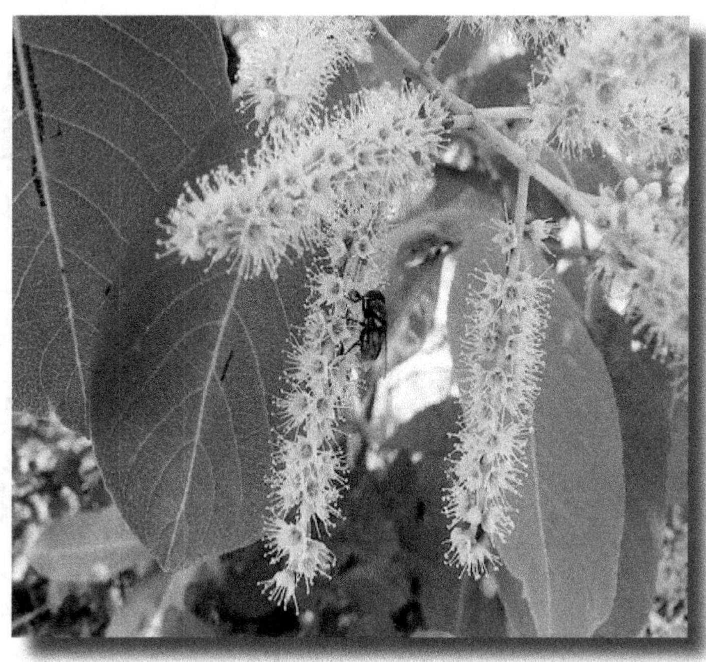

In Indian mythology, Arjun is supposed to be Sita's favourite tree. Native to India, the tree attracts lot of attention because of its association with mythology and its many uses. Arjuna is a large, evergreen tree, with a spreading crown and drooping branches. Grows up to 25 m height, and the bark is grey and smooth. Leaves are sub-opposite, 5-14 × 2-4.5 cm in size, oblong or elliptic oblong. Flowers small, white, and occur on long hanging recemes. Fruit is 2.3-3.5 cm long, fibrous woody, glabrous and has five hard wings, striated with numerous curved veins. Flowering time of the tree is April-July, in Indian conditions.

Medicinal Uses:

Every part of the tree has useful medicinal properties. Arjun holds a reputed position in both *Ayurvedic and Yunani Systems of medicine.* According to Ayurveda, it is *alexiteric, styptic, tonic, anthelmintic, and useful in fractures, uclers, heart diseases, biliousness, urinary discharges, asthma, tumours, leucoderma, anaemia, excessive prespiration,* etc. According to the Yunani system of medicine, it is used both externally and internally in *gleet and urinary discharges.*

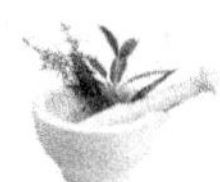

Baheda

Botanical Name:

Terminalia bellirica

Family:

Combretaceae (**Rangoon creeper family**)

Synonyms:

Myrobalanus bellirica

Common Names:

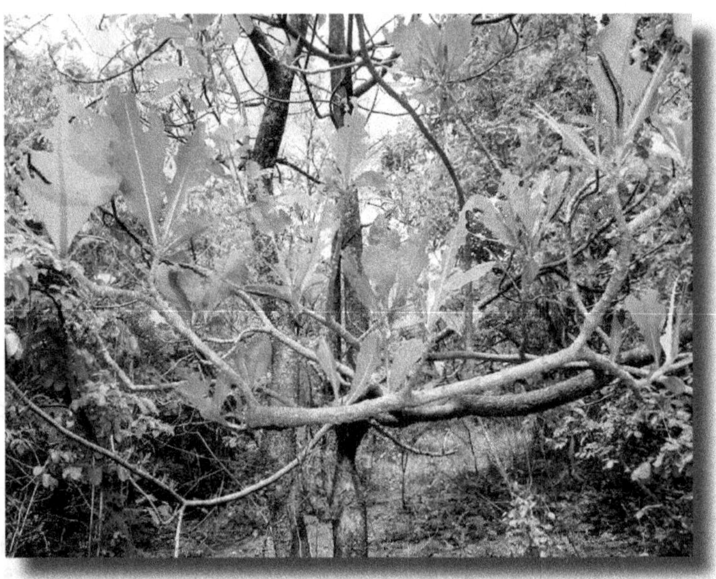

Baheda, Belliric Myrobalan, Bastard myrobalan, Beach almond, Bedda nut tree • Hindi: *Bahera, Bahuvirya, Bhutvaas, Kalk, Karshphal* • Manipuri: *Bahera* • Marathi: *Behada, Bibh,taka, Kalidruma, Vehala* • Tamil: *Tanri* • Malayalam: *Thaanni* • Telugu: *Bhutavasamu, Karshaphalamu, Tadi, Tandrachettu, Vibhitakamu* • Kannada: *Taarekaayi* • Bengali: *Baheda* • Oriya: *Bahada* • Konkani: *Goting* • Urdu: *Bahera* • Assamese: *Bauri* • Gujarati: *Baheda* • Khasi: *Dieng rinyn* • Sanskrit: *Akshah, Bahuvirya, Bibhitakah, Karshah, Vibhitakah* • Nepali: *Barro*

Description:

Baheda is a tall handsome tree, with characteristic bark, 12-50 m tall. Leaves are alternately arranged or fascicled at the end of branches, elliptic or elliptic obovate, leathery, dotted, entire. Leaf tip is narrow-pointed or rounded. Leaves are 8-20 cm long, 7.5-15 cm wide, on stalks 2.15 cm long. Flowers arise in spikes in leaf axils, 5-15 cm long. Flowers are greenish yellow, 5-6 mm across, stalklesse, upper flowers of the spike are male, lower flowers are bisexual. Stamens are 3-4 mm long. Fruit is obovoid 1.5-2.5 cm in diameter, covered with minute pale pubescence, stone very thick, indistinctly 5 angled.

Medicinal Uses:

In traditional *Indian Ayurvedic medicine*, Baheda is known as 'Bibhitaki' in its fruit form, and is used in the popular *Indian herbal rasayana treatment, triphala*. This species is used by some tribes in the Indian subcontinent for its mind-altering qualities - they smoke *dried kernels*. However, too much of this can *cause nausea* and *vomiting*.

Chebulic Myrobalan

Botanical Name:

Terminalia chebula

Family:

Combretaceae (**Rangoon creeper family**)

Common Names:

Chebulic Myrobalan, Myrobalan • Hindi: *Harra, Harad* • Manipuri: *Manahi* • Marathi: *Hirad* • Tamil: *Kadukkaay* • Malayalam: *Katukka* • Telugu: *Nallakaraka* • Kannada: *Halle* • Bengali: *Haritaki* • Oriya: *Karedha* • Konkani: *Ordo* • Assamese: *Hilika* • Sanskrit: *Kayastha, Jivapriya*

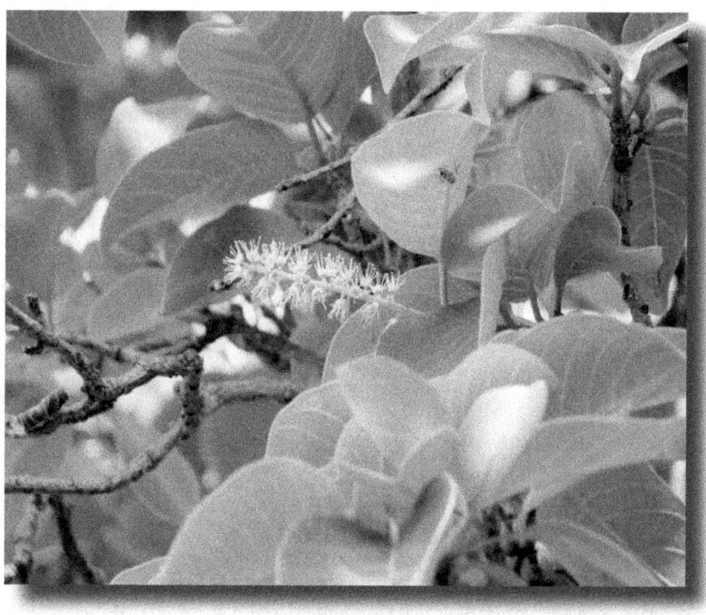

Description:

Chebulic Myrobalan is a flowering evergreen tree called in English the Myrobalan or sometimes the Chebulic Myrobalan. It is native to the Indian subcontinent and the adjacent areas such as Pakistan, Nepal and the south-west of China stretching as far south as Kerala or even Sri Lanka where is called Aralu. This tree yields smallish, ribbed and nut-like fruits which are picked up when still green and then pickled, boiled with a little added sugar in their own syrup or used in preserves or concotions. The seed of the fruit, which has an eliptical shape, is an abrasive pit enveloped by a fleshy and firm pulp. *Chebulic Myrobalan can reach heights of about 20 metres.*

Medicinal Uses:

Chebulic Myrobalan is highly regarded as the '*king of medicines*' in the *Ayurvedic Medicine*. It is *reputed to cure blindness* and is believed to *inhibit the growth of malignant tumours*. It is allegedly also a *powerful detox agent.*

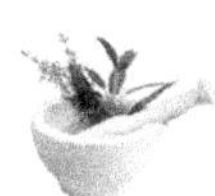

"

Grass of the Dew

Botanical Name:

Cyanotis arachnoidea

Family:

Commelinaceae (**Dayflower family**)

Synonyms:

Cyanotis bodinieri

Common Names:

Grass of the Dew

Description:

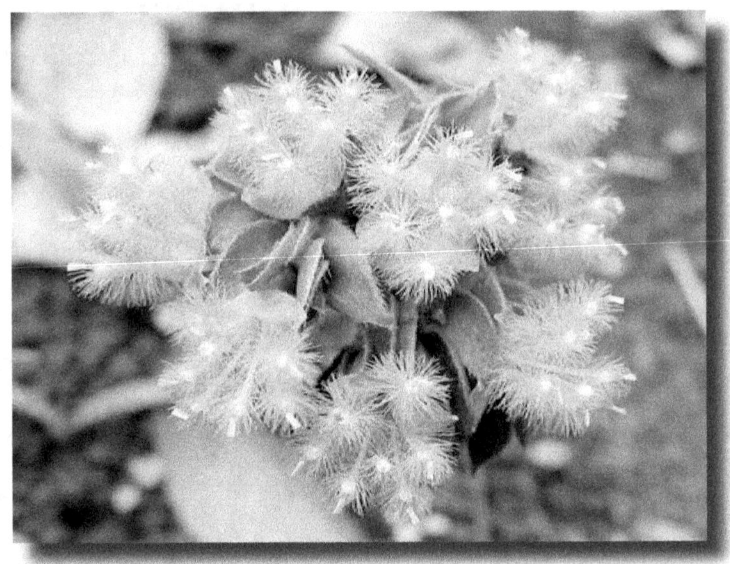

Grass of the Dew plant has furry violet blooms, dotted with yellow stamens. It is a perennial her with fibrous roots. Main stem is undeveloped, short. Fertile stems arise from below the leaf rosette, diffuse, creeping, 20-80 cm. Leaves are in a basal rosette and cauline. Rosulate leaf blade linear, 8-35 × 0.5-1.5 cm; cauline leaf blade on fertile stems much shorter, to 7 cm, abaxially rather densely arachnoid. Flowers arise in often several, both terminal and axillary heads, stalkless or on a stalk up to 4 cm. Bracts are 7-8 mm. Sepals are fused at base, linear-lanceshaped, about 5 mm, webby on the underside. Petals are blue-purple, blue, or white, about 6 mm. Filaments are blue, cobweb-like. Capsules are broadly oblong, trigonous, about 2.5 mm, densely hairy at the tip. Flowering: June–September.

Medicinal Uses:

The Grass of the Dew was used to cure *rheumatic infections* in the China Imperial. The *roots* are used as medicine for *stimulating blood circulation*, as a *muscle and joint relaxant*, and for *relieving rheumatoid arthritis*.

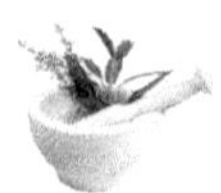

Rudravanti

Botanical Name:
Cressa cretica

Family:
Convolvulaceae (**Morning glory family**)

Common Names:
Rudravanti, Littoral bind weed • Hindi: *Rudravanti* • Marathi: *Lona, Rudravanti* • Tamil: *Uppucanaka* • Malayalam: *Azhukanni* • Telugu: *Uppugaddi, Uppusenaga* • Kannada: *Mullumaddugida* • Konkani: *Chaval* • Urdu: *Rudanti* • Gujarati: *Una* • Sanskrit: *Rudravanti, Palitaka*

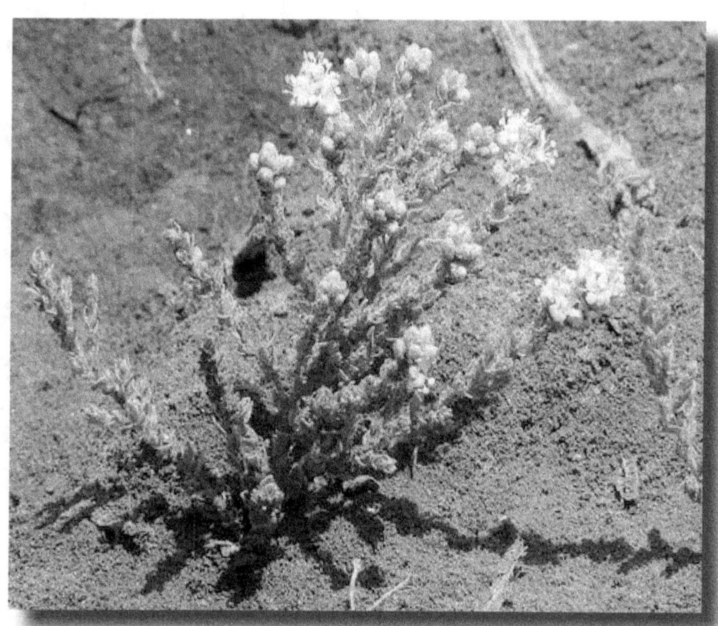

Description:
Rudravanti is a shrubby, diffused herb, a few cm to 30 cm high, arising from a woody perennial root-stock. It is commonly found in India along sandy sea shores. Numerous stalkless leaves are very small, ovate, acute tipped, hairy or ashy-velvety. Flowers are small, white or pink, nearly stalkless in upper leaf axils, forming a many-flowered head. Sepals are 5, flower is funnel-shaped, and stamens protrude out of the flower. It is commonly in cultivated fields about Mumbai. Flowering: December-February.

Medicinal Uses:
According to Ayurveda, it is *bitter, pungent, rough and hot in properties.* The *whole plant* is used for *medicinal purposes.* It is a useful herb for *asthma, bronchitis, dyspepsia, flatulence, colic, anorexia, anaemia, diabetes* and *skin diseases.*

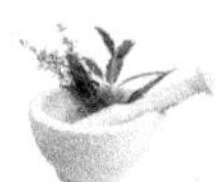

Dwarf Morning Glory

Botanical Name:
Evolvulus alsinoides

Family:
Convolvulaceae (**Morning glory family**)

Common Names:
Dwarf Morning Glory, Slender Dwarf Morning Glory • Hindi: *Visnukrantha, Shyamakrantha* • Marathi: *Vishnukranta* • Tamil: *Vishnukranthi* • Malayalam: *Vishnukranthi* • Telugu: *Vishnukrantha* • Kannada: *Vishnykranti* • Sanskrit: *Vishnugandhi*

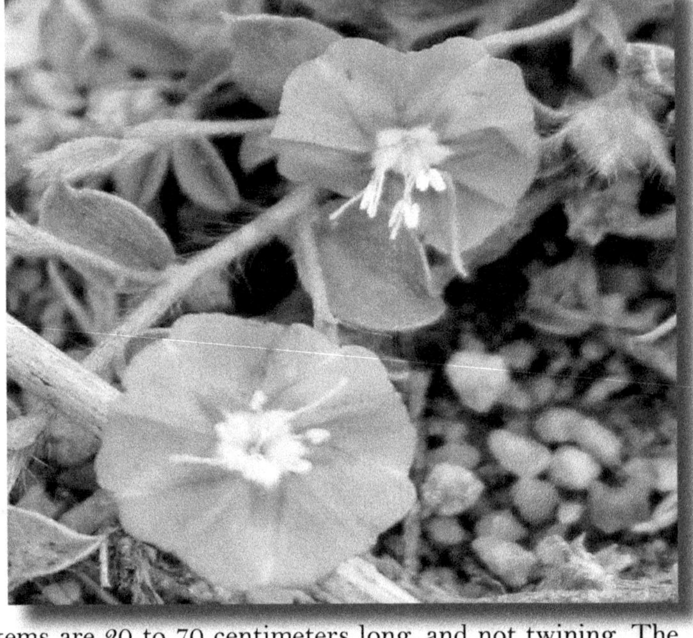

Description:
This is a very slender, more or less branched, spreading or ascending, usually extremely hairy herb. The stems are 20 to 70 centimeters long, and not twining. The leaves, which are densely clothed with appressed, white, and silky hairs, are variable clothed, lanceolate to ovate, and usually 0.5 to 1 centimetre (cm) in length (but may be larger); the apex is blunt with a little point and the base is pointed. The flowers are pale blue and 6-8 mm in diameter. The fruit (capsule) is rounded, and usually contains four seeds.

Medicinal Uses:
The whole plant is used in the Goa territory. It is used extensively as *a febrifuge* and *tonic. With cumin and milk*, it is used for *fevers nervous debility* and *loss of memory*, and also for *syphilis, scrofula*, etc. it is said to be a sovereign remedy for *bowel complaints*, especially *dysentery*.

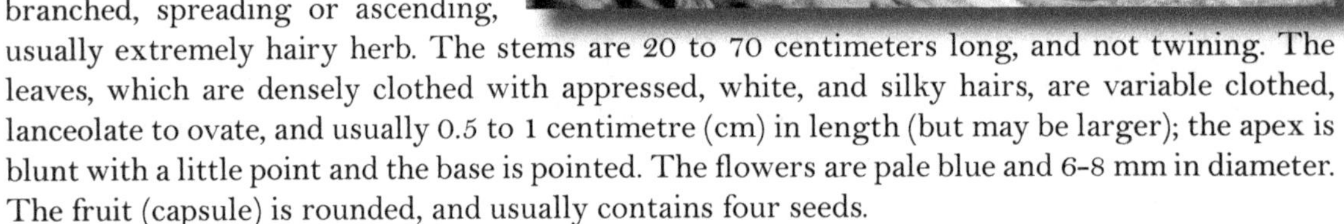

Giant Potato

Botanical Name:

Ipomoea mauritiana

Family:

Convolvulaceae (**Morning glory family**)

Synonyms:

Ipomoea digitata, Ipomoea insignis

Common Names:

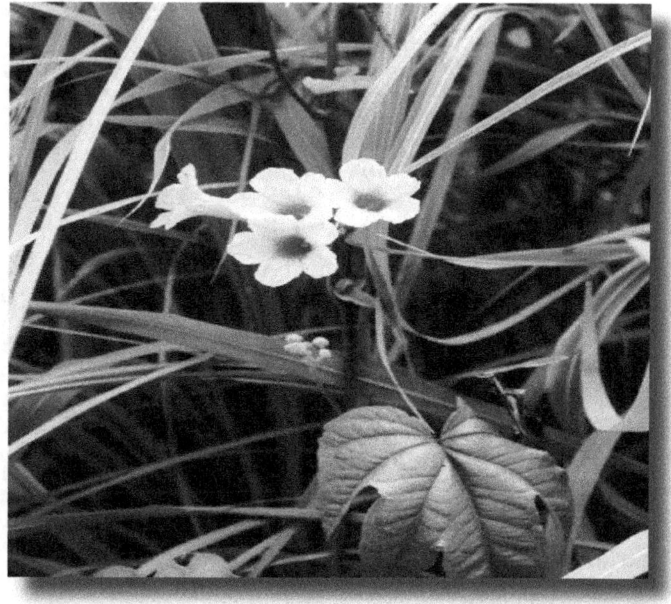

Giant potato, Large Forest Ipomoea • Hindi: *Bhuyikohada* • Telugu: *Nelagummudu* • Tamil: *Palmudamgi* • Malayalam: *Mutalakkilannu* • Marathi: *Bhui-kohala*

Description:

The Giant Potato is a type of morning glory plant. Like the sweet potato, it belongs to the Ipomoea genera. It grows as a vine. The origin of Ipomoea mauritiana is unknown, it is there all over the tropics. It is naturalised in many parts of the world. This vine has stems that can grow to 10 m. Leaf blade is circular in outline, 7-18 X 7-22 cm, usually palmately 5-7-divided to or beyond middle, rarely entire or shallowly lobed. Inflorescences few to many flowered. Flowers are pink or reddish purple, with a darker centre, funnelform, 5-6 cm across.

Medicinal Uses:

The leaves and roots are used *externally* to *treat tuberculosis* and for the *treatment of external and breast infections.* In Ayurveda, a *decoction of the tuberous roots* are used for the preparation of *medicinal wine.* The Ayurvedic Name is *Kiribadu Ala,* and it is also an ingredient in the popular, *Chyavanprash.*

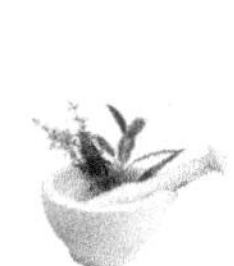

Kidney Leaf Morning Glory

Botanical Name:

Merremia gangetica

Family:

Convolvulaceae (**Morning glory family**)

Synonyms:

Merremia emarginata, Convolvulus reniformis, Ipomoea reniformis

Common Names:

Kidney Leaf Morning Glory • Hindi: *Musakani* • Marathi: *Undirkani* • Tamil: *Elikkadhu-keerai* • Telugu: *Elikajemudu*

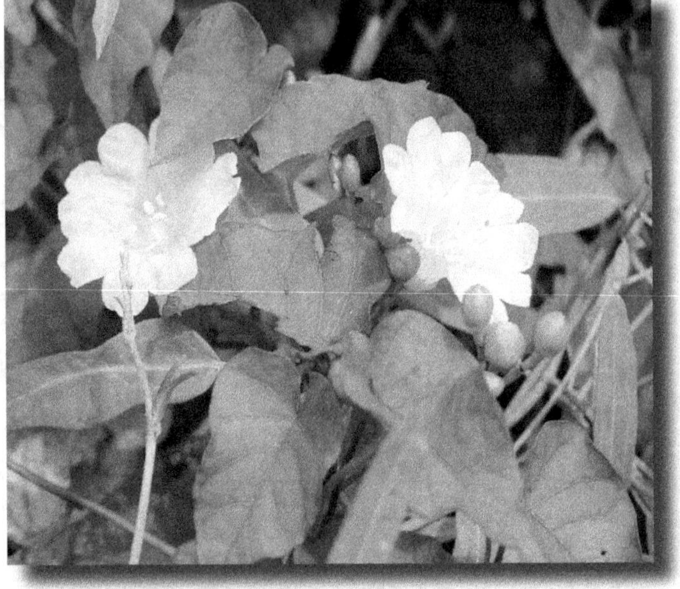

Description:

This is a slender, prostates, creeping, smooth or somewhat hairy herb. The stems root at the nodes, and are 10-80 cm in length. The leaves are small, kidney-shaped to somewhat heart-shaped, 6-15 mm long, often wider than long, and irregularly toothed. One to three flowers occur on short stalks in the axils of the leaves. The sepals are rounded and about 4 mm long, with few to many white, weak hairs. The corolla is yellow, and nearly twice as long as the calyx. The capsule is rounded and about 5 mm in diameter.

Medicinal Uses:

In the Philippines, the *decocted leaves and tops* are sometimes employed as a *diuretic*. In India, the leaves are useful as a *diuretic* and an *alterative* and are also used in *rheumatism* and *neuralgia*.

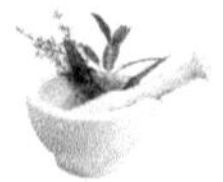

Painted Spiral Ginger

Botanical Name:
Costus pictus

Family:
Costaceae (**Spiral Ginger family**)

Synonyms:
Costus hieroglyphica, Costus mexicanus, Costus congestus

Common Names:
Painted Spiral Ginger, Spotted Spiral Ginger

Description:
Painted Spiral Ginger is a perennial herb, native to Mexico. It has long narrow leaves with a

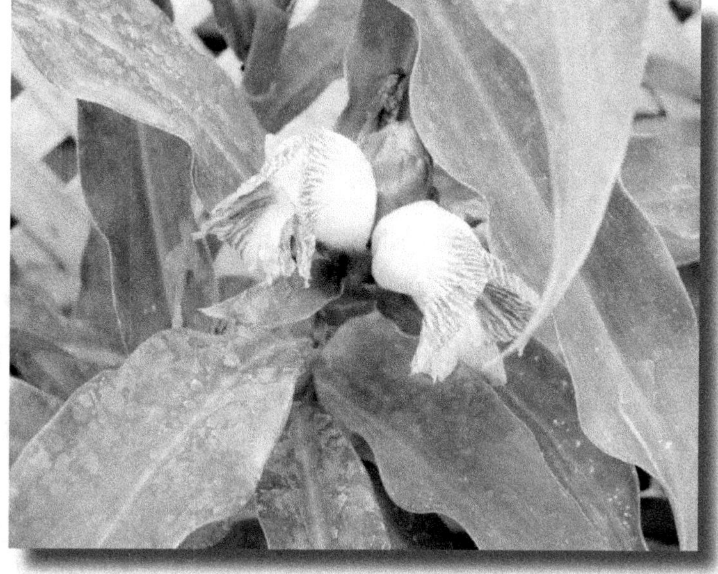

characteristic wavy edges. The bases of the sheaths are mottled with markings that have earned the plant the synonym of Costus hieroglyphica. The inflorescences form both at the end of a leafy stem, and less often radically on a short nearly leafless stem. Painted Spiral Ginger can be recognized by its yellow flowers with red spots and stripes. In India it is grown in gardens as orNamental plant especially in Kerala in every home. The major attraction of this plant is its stem with spiral leaves and light airy and tissue paper like flowers. Red painted stem enhances the beauty of the glossy leaves and strongly spiralling canes.

Medicinal Uses:
The *Costus pictus* is valued mainly for its *tonic, stimulant* and *antiseptic properties*. It is said to be *aphrodisiac* and to be able to prevent *the hair turning grey*. Its *root* is *anodyne, antibacterial, antispasmodic, aphrodisiac, carminative*, skin-stimulant, stomachic, tonic and vermifuge.

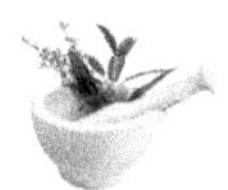

Air Plant

Botanical Name:

Kalanchoe pinnata/ Bryophyllum pinnatum

Family:

Crassulaceae (**Sedum family**)

Common Names:

Air Plant, Donkey Ears, Life Plant, Leaf of Life, Resurrection Plant, Canterbury Bells, Cathedral Bells, Mexican Love Plant, Floppers • Hindi: *Amar poi* • Malayalam: *Elamarunna* • Tamil: *Runakkalli* • Bengali: *Kop pata* • Urdu: *Zakhmhaiyat* • Manipuri: *Manahidak*

Description:

It is a native Hawaiian plant. Easy to grow just from one leaf set on top of moist soil. Very fast growing, drought tolerant small shrub. Tolerates almost any conditions. Spectacular bloomer. Air Plant grows to about 3-6 feet tall. The erect, thick, succulent stems bear large, fleshy leaves, each with 3 or 5 oval leaflets with round-toothed edges. Young plantlets develop along the margins of the mature leaves. The attractive, drooping blooms are borne on large panicles. The flowers have purple or yellowish-white tinged calyxes and reddish corollas. Kalanchoe is a genus of about 125 species of tropical, succulent flowering plants in the Family Crassulaceae, mainly native to the Old World but with a few species in the New World. These plants are cultivated as orNamental houseplants and rock or "cactus" garden plants. They are popular because of their ease of propagation, low water requirements, and wide variety of flower colours typically borne in clusters well above the vegetative growth. The "Air plant" Kalanchoe pinnata is a curiosity because new individuals develop vegetatively at indents along the leaf, usually after the leaf has broken off the plant and is laying on the ground, where the new plant can take root.

Medicinal Uses:

The Bahamians call it as *Life Leaf* or *Ploppers*. In the Bahamas, it is mostly used for *asthma* or *shortness* in *breath*.

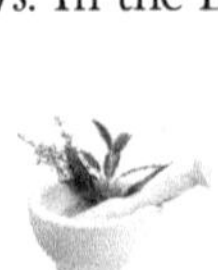

Chinese Cucumber

Botanical Name:

Momordica cochinchinensis

Family:

Cucurbitaceae (**Pumpkin family**)

Common Names:

Chinese Cucumber, Spiny bitter-cucumber, Chinese bitter-cucumber • Hindi: *Kakur, Kantola, Kakrol* • Manipuri: *Karot* • Marathi: *Gulkakra* • Malayalam: *Kshudramalakasanda* • Telugu: *Varivalli* • Bengali: *Golkakra* • Assamese: *Bhat kerala* • Sanskrit: *Katamala*

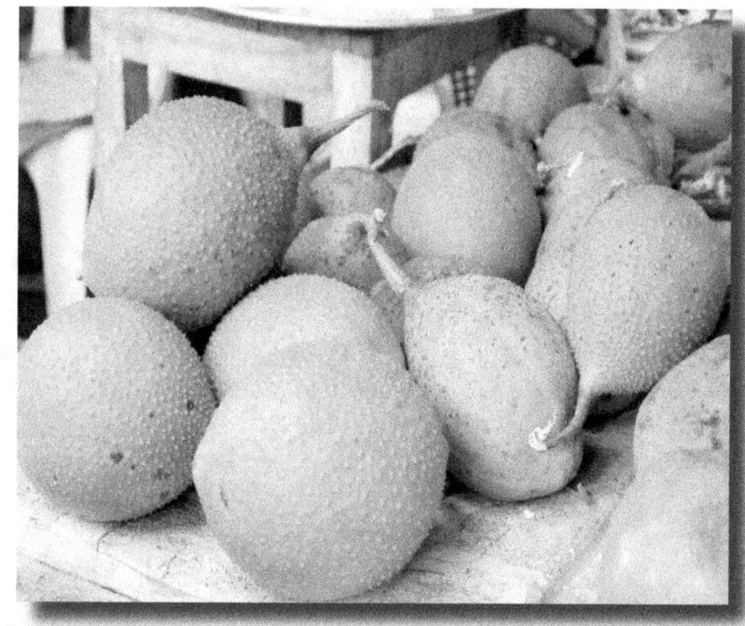

Description:

Chinese cucumber is a traditional medicinal plant in India, China and Vietnam, commonly seen growing in gardens with its red fruit and red pulp. It is found throughout Asia and Australia. It is used in cooking, to make candy and jam, and is thought to support the health of the eyes. Aril, the red, oily pulp surrounding the seeds, is cooked along with seeds to flavour and give its red colour to a rice dish, xoi gac, which is served at festive occasions such as weddings in Vietnam. It has large leaves and large white flowers.

Medicinal Uses:

The seeds are used in *Ayurvedic* and *Chinese traditional medicine*. The total content of *beta-carotene* in this *fruit* is very high, which is definitely good for the skin and eyes.

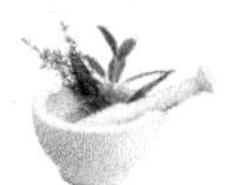

Wild Cucumber

Botanical Name:
Zehneria scabra

Family:
Cucurbitaceae (**Pumpkin family**)

Synonyms:
Melothria perpusilla

Common Names:
Wild Cucumber, South African zehneria, Cape zehneria • Manipuri: *Lam thabi* • Marathi: *Chirati* • Tamil: *Naai pagal*

Description:
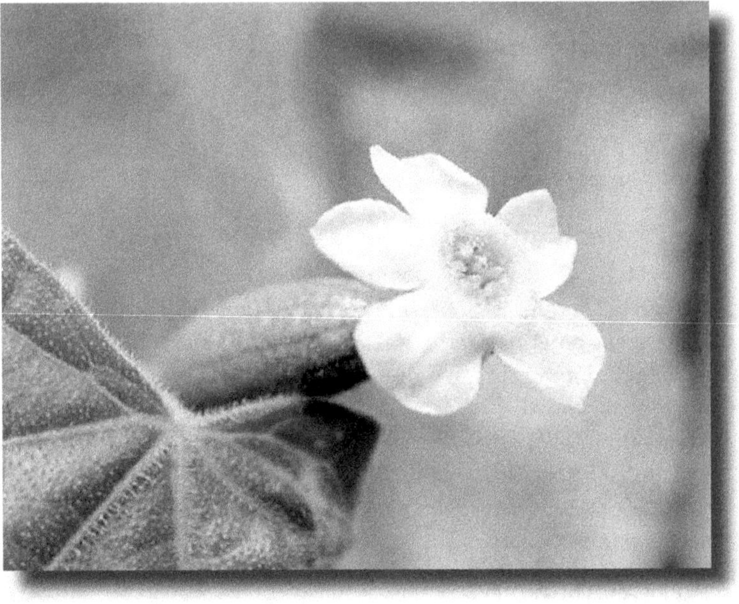

Wild Cucumber is a perennial climber which climbs using tendrils. Leaves are heart-shaped and lobed, with distant spiny teeth on the margin. Flowers are small, white. Fruits look like miniature watermelons, and taste like cucumber. This species is a bit difficult to distinguish from Zehneria maysorensis, which is a native.

Medicinal Uses:
The plant is useful in *the treatment of jaundice* and *kidney infections* other *than stones*. In *kidney problems*, the *boiled decoction of the shoots of the plant* and the *Touch Me Not* in equal proportions, mixed with *molasses is prescribed as a remedy.*

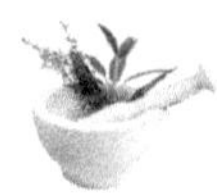

"/>

Umbrella Sedge

Botanical Name:
Cyperus scariosus

Family:
Cyperaceae (**Sedge family**)

Common Names:
Umbrella Sedge, Nutgrass, Nutsedge, Purple Nutsedge • Hindi: *Nagarmotha* • Marathi: *Lawala* • Tamil: *Koraikkilangu, Nakamuttakkacu* • Malayalam: *Korakizhanna* • Telugu: *Kolatungamuste, Tungagaddalaveru* • Kannada: *Konnarigadda, Nagarmusthe* • Urdu: *Nagarmotha, Sadkofi* • Sanskrit: *Chakranksha, Charukesara, Chudalapindamusta, Kachharuha, Kalapini, Nadeyi, Nagar-mustaka*

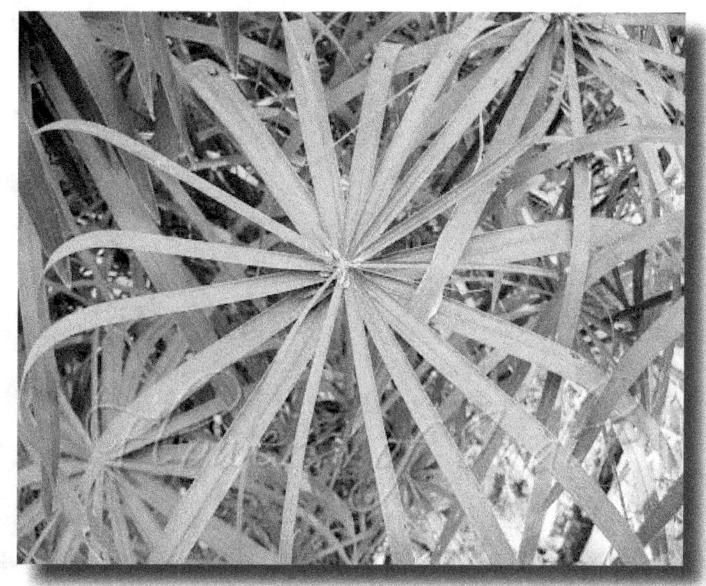

Description:
Umbrella Sedge is a perennial herb, about a meter tall, arising from rhizomes and tubers. The stems are 3-sided and triangular in cross section and there is an umbrella-like tuft of long narrow leaves at the top. The leaves are yellow to green in colour with a distinct ridge. The plant has red-brown flower spikelets with up to 40 individual flowers. The dried tuberous roots are collected, dried and used in traditional medicine. Nutgrass is used in hair - and skin care products. It stimulates sebaceous glands near hair roots. Also interesting is that the oil, an amber viscous liquid, extracted from this plant is used in perfumery.

Medicinal Uses:
The tubers are credited with *astringent, diaphoretic, diuretic, dessicant, cordial and stomachic* properties. A *decoction of the tuber* is used for *washing hair*, treating *gonorrhoea* and *syphilis*. It is also given in diarrhoea and for *general weakness*.

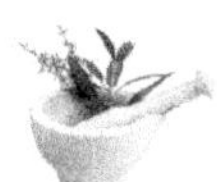

Karmal

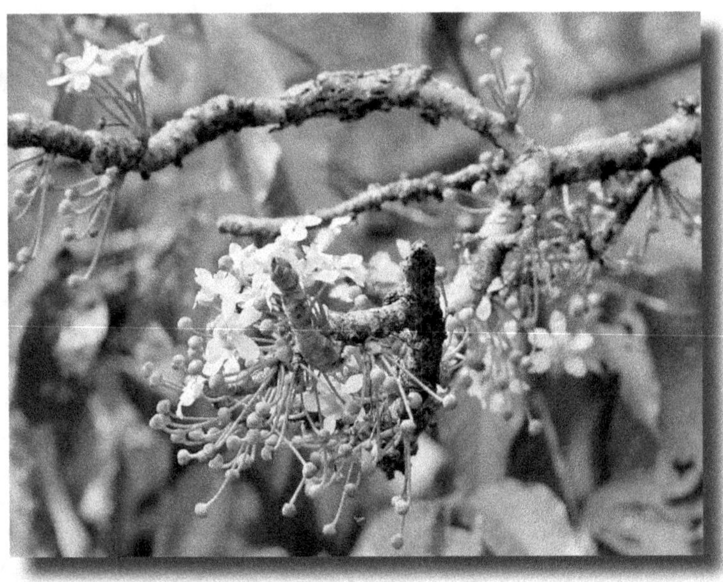

Botanical Name:
Dillenia pentagyna

Family:
Dilleniaceae (**Karmal family**)

Synonyms:
Dillenia floribunda, Dillenia hainanensis

Common Names:
Karmal, Dog Teak, Dillenia, Nepali elephant apple • Hindi: *Karmal* • Marathi: *Piwala karmal* • Tamil: *Nay-t-tekku, Punnai vakai* • Malayalam: *Kutapunna, Pattippunna, Vaazhappunna* • Telugu: *Chinna kalinga, Revada* • Kannada: *Kaadu kanigalu* • Bengali: *Ban chalta* • Oriya: *Railgatcho* • Konkani: *Lahan karmal* • Assamese: *Okshi* • Gujarati: *Karmal* • Khasi: *Dieng soh bar* • Mizo: *Kaihzawl, Kawrthing-dengte* • Sanskrit: *Aksikiphal, Punnaga* • Nepalese: *Ram phal, Tantari*

Description:
Karmal is a large deciduous tree grows up to 40 meters in height. Leaves are large, 1-2 ft, alternate, ovate-rhomboid, obtuse or acute. Flowers yellowish, fragrant, 2-3 cm across, arise from the nodes of fallen leaves, on panicles. Fruits 2.5 cm in diameter, globose contain single seed. The flower-buds and young fruits have a pleasant, acid flavour and are eaten raw or cooked in Oudh and central India. The ripe fruits are also eaten. Dillenia, Named in honour of J. J. Dillenius (1684–1747), a noted botanist. Pentagyna in allusion to the flower having five styles. Flowering: March-May.

Medicinal Uses:
According to *Ayurveda*, the plant pacifies *vitiated vata, kapha, anal fistula, wounds, diabetes, diabetic carbuncle, neuritis, pleurisy, pneumonia* and *burning sensations*.

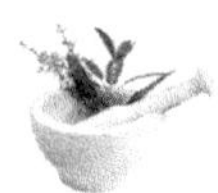

Wild Yam

Botanical Name:
Dioscorea villosa

Family:
Dioscoreaceae (**Yam family**)

Synonyms:
Dioscorea glauca, Dioscorea hirticaulis, Dioscorea quaternata

Common Names:
Wild Yam, Colic Root

Description:
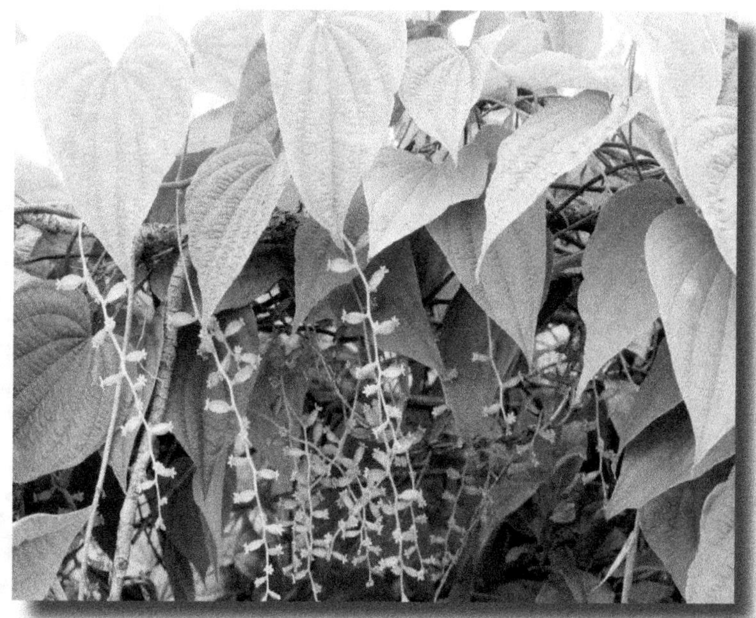

Native to North America, Wild Yam is a perennial vine which can reach a height of 10 ft. The stem is slender, rarely branched and tends to twine right to left or counterclockwise. Alternately arranged leaves are heart- shaped. The lowest leaves may appear whorled. Leaves have 7-11 parallel veins, and may be hairy on the underside. Wild yam has separate male and female flowers, yellow-green, in loose straggling clusters. Female flowers sit on top of winged green fruits. Flowering time: June–August.

Medicinal Uses:

The native Americans and early herbalists had many uses of this plant including the treatment of many *female and childbirth related problems*. It was also used to treat various *gastrointestinal problems, muscle spasms, various painful conditions*, such as *arthritis* and *rheumatism*. There seems to be no scientific evidence of its effectiveness for these conditions. Nonetheless, plants of this genus are valuable to *modern medicine*. Many of *our modern steroids* are manufactured from *diosgenin* extracted from them.

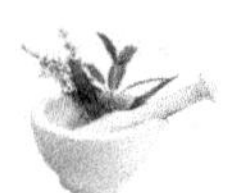

Gaub

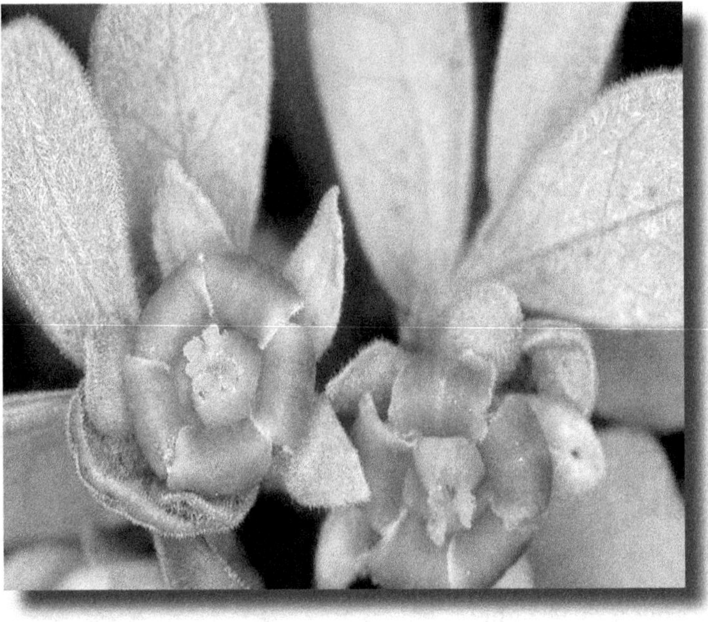

Botanical Name:

Diospyros malabarica

Family:

Ebenaceae (**Ebony family**)

Synonyms:

Diospyros peregrine

Common Names:

Hindi: *Gaub* • Tamil: *Tumbika* • Marathi: *Temburi* • Malayalam: *Panancca* • Telugu: *Bandadamara* • Kannada: *Holitupare*

Description:

Gab is an *evergreen tree* with a *spreading crown.* The leaves are long and glossy. The flowers have a tough texture and are creamish in colour, in clusters of 3-6.

Medicinal Uses:

Gab is the *Tinduka* of Sanskrit writers; its bark is described in the *Nighantas* as a good application to *boils* and *tumours,* and the juice of the fresh bark is useful in *bilious fever.* The fruit when unripe is said to be *cold, light* and *astringent,* and when ripe, it is beneficial in *blood diseases, gonorrhoea* and *leprosy.*

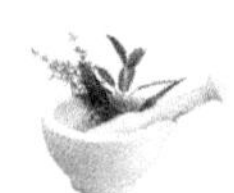

Jamaica Cherry

Botanical Name:
Muntingia calabura

Family:
Elaeocarpaceae (**Rudraksh family**)

Common Names:
Jamaica Cherry, Panama Cherry, Strawberry tree, Jam tree, Cotton Candy berry, Calabura • Marathi: *Paanchara* • Tamil: *Ten pazham* • Telugu: *Nakkaraegu* • Kannada: *Gasagase hannina mara*

Description:

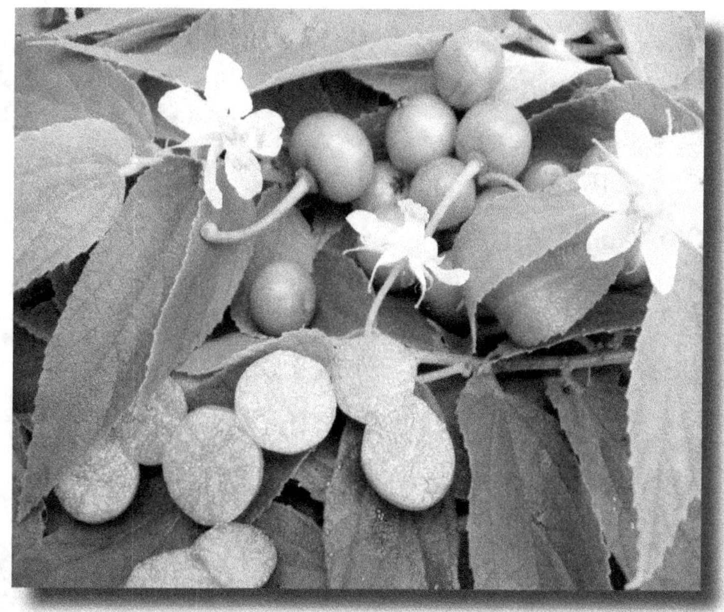

Jamaica Cherry is a very fast-growing tree of slender proportions, reaching 25 to 40 ft in height, with spreading, nearly horizontal branches. The leaves are evergreen, alternate, lanceolate or oblong, long-pointed at the apex, oblique at the base. The flowers with 5 green sepals and 5 white petals and many prominent yellow stamens last only one day, the petals falling in the afternoon. Flowers resemble strawberry bloom, hence the common Name, Strawberry tree. The abundant fruits are round, 1-1.25 cm wide, with red or sometimes yellow, smooth, thin, tender skin and light-brown, soft, juicy pulp, with very sweet, musky, somewhat fig-like flavour, filled with exceedingly minute, yellowish seeds, too fine to be noticed in eating. The tree has the reputation of thriving with no care in poor soils. It is drought-resistant but not salt-tolerant. Wherever it grows, fruits are borne nearly all year. The leaf infusion is drunk as a tea-like beverage. Fruits contain hundreds of tiny seeds.

Medicinal Uses:

The flowers are said to possess *antiseptic properties*. An infusion of the flowers is valued as an *antispasmodic*. It is taken to relieve headaches and the first symptoms of a *cold*.

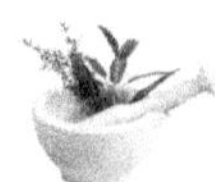

Dwarf Rhododendron

Botanical Name:
Rhododendron anthopogon

Family:
Ericaceae **(Rhododendron family)**

Common Names:
Dwarf Rhododendron, Hindi: *Talis, Talisri*

Description:
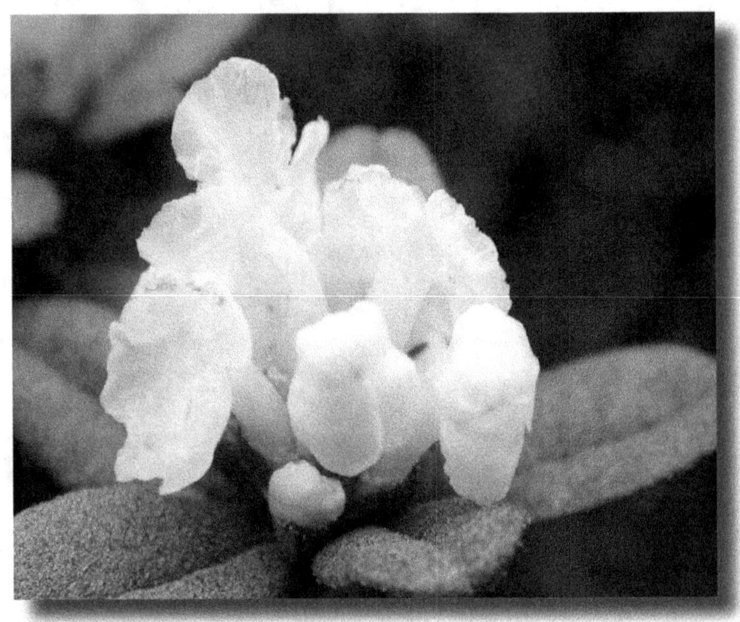

This is probably one of the smallest of rhododendrons. Grows to no more that 2-3 ft high. The white or yellow flowers, tinged with pink, grow in small compact clusters of 4-6 and each flower is 2 cm across. The dark green oval leaves are strongly aromatic and densely scaly underneath. The leaves are mixed with Juniper and used as incense in Buddhist monasteries as well as in Hindu religious ceremonies.

Medicinal Uses:

In Nepal, *Dwarf Rhododendron* is used in making an *essential oil*. The *Anthopogon oil*, as it is usually referred to in Nepal, is obtained by *steam distillation* of the *aerial part of this shrub*. It is a fluid liquid of pale yellow colour and sweet-herbal, faintly balsamic aroma. The Rhododendron can be used in *gouty rheumatic conditions*. The essential oil is a *stimulant* and affects the fibrous tissues, *bones* and the *nervous system*.

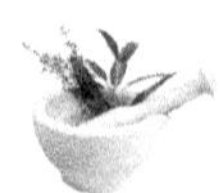

Pink Scaly Rhododendron

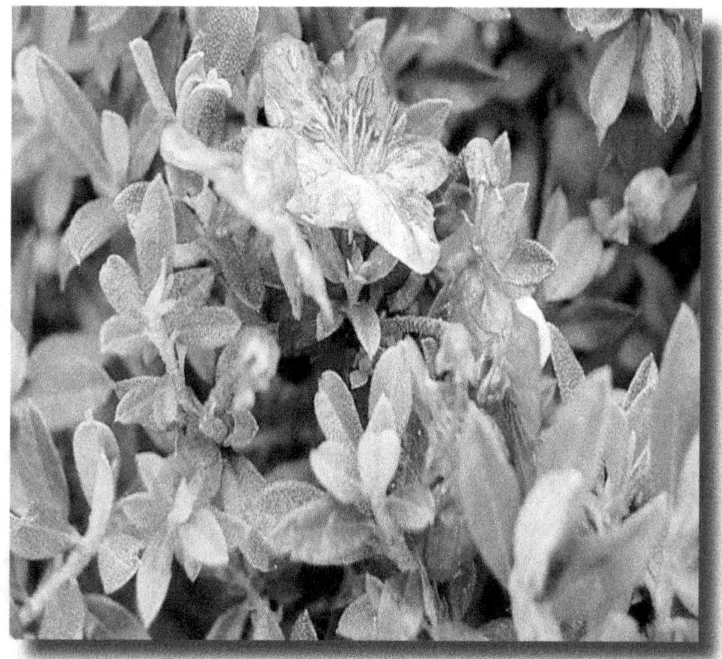

Botanical Name:

Rhododendron lepidotum

Family:

Ericaceae (**Rhododendron family**)

Common Names:

Pink Scaly Rhododendron • Hindi: *Atarasu, Sumral, Simris, Talshi* • Nepali: *Bhaale Sunpati*

Description:

Pink Scaly Rhododendron is a low shrublet, growing to about a meter tall. Narrow lanceshaped leaves, 2.5-4 cm long, are densely covered with fleshy scales. Flowers are pink or purple, borne in clusters of 2 to 4, on slender stalks. Flowers are about 2-2.5 cm across, broadly tubular with 5 spreading rounded petals, scaly and glandular outside. Eight stamens protrude out of the flowers with red filaments which are hairy on the lower side. Fruit is a capsule, densely scaly, covered with persisting sepals. Flowering: June-July.

Medicinal Uses:

The people of Manang district, central Nepal, take the juice of the plant, believing it *purifies the blood. Pounded leaves are boiled in water* and spread *on cots, beds and mats* to *kill bugs.*

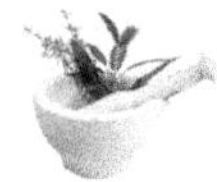

Yellow Scaly Rhododendron

Botanical Name:
Rhododendron lepidotum ssp. salignum

Family:
Ericaceae (**Rhododendron family**)

Synonyms:
Rhododendron salignum

Common Names:
Yellow Scaly Rhododendron • Hindi: *Atarasu, Sumral, Simris, Talshi* • Nepali: *Bhaale Sunpati*

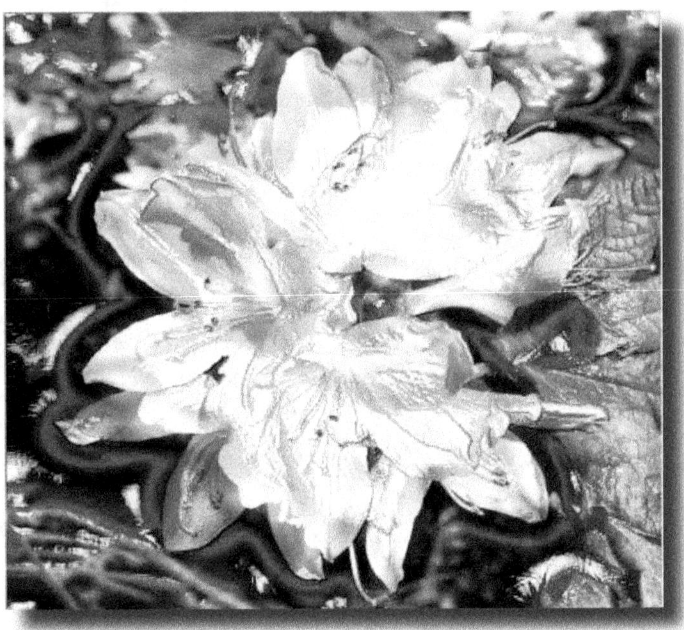

Description:
Yellow Scaly Rhododendron is a low shrublet, growing to about a meter tall. Narrow lanceshaped leaves, 2.5-4 cm long, are densely covered with fleshy scales. Flowers are pale yellow, borne in clusters of 2 to 4, on slender stalks. Flowers are about 2-2.5 cm across, broadly tubular with 5 spreading rounded petals, scaly and glandular outside. Eight stamens protrude out of the flowers with filaments which are hairy on the lower side. Fruit is a capsule, densely scaly, covered with persisting sepals. Flowering: June–July.

Medicinal Uses:
The people of the Manang district, central Nepal take the juice of the plant, believing it *purifies the blood. Pounded leaves are boiled in water* and spread on *cots, beds and mats* to *kill bugs.*

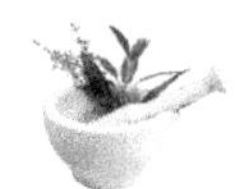

Red Physic Nut

Botanical Name:

Baliospermum montanum

Family:

Euphorbiaceae (**Castor family**)

Synonyms:

Baliospermum axillare, Baliospermum solanifolium, Jatropha Montana

Common Names:

Red Physic Nut, Wild castor, Wild croton, Wild sultan seed • Hindi: *Danti* • Marathi: *Danti, Katari* • Tamil: *Pey-amanakku* • Malayalam: *Ceriyadanthi, Naagadanthi* • Telugu: *Adavi amudamu, Kond amudamu, Nela jidi, Nepalamu* •

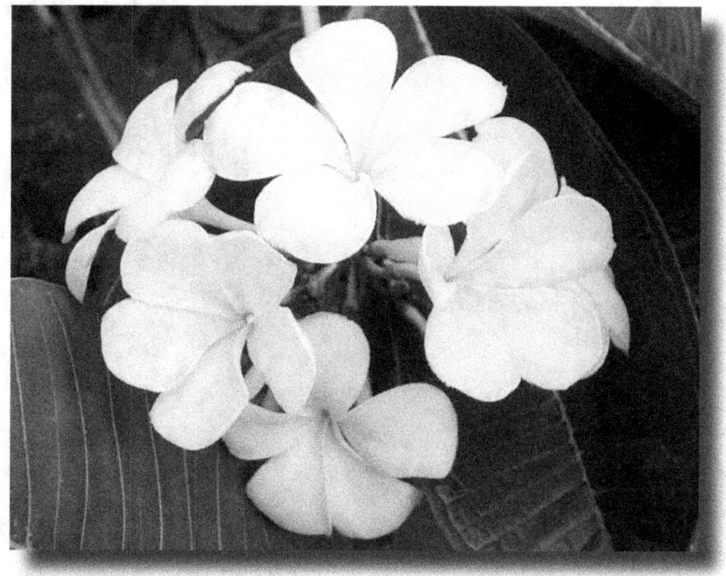

Kannada: *Damti, Kaadu haralu, Naagadamti* • Bengali: *Danti, Dantigaacha* • Konkani: *Baktumbo* • Sanskrit: *Danti, Dantika, Dirgha, Erandhapatrika, Erandhaphala, Makulakah, Nagadanti, Nagavinna, Nikumbha, Pratyaksreni, Rechani, Ruksha, Shigra, Vishalya, Udumbaraparni* • Nepali: *Ajaya pal, Dudhe Jhaar*

Description:

Red Physic Nut is a stout undershrub, 10 cm to 8 m in height with herbaceous branches from the roots. Leaves are simple, toothed with undulations. Upper leaves are small, lower ones large, sometimes palmately 3-5 lobed, 3-30 cm long, 1.5-15 cm broad. Male and female flowers are separated, seen in the same flowering branch, minute, about 3 mm across, greenish yellow, arranged in axillary and terminal racemes, spikes or fascicles. Capsules are distinctly 3-lobed, obovoid, stony, 8-13 mm across, minutely densely pubescent. Seeds are egg-shaped.

Medicinal Uses:

Roots, seeds, leaves and seed oil are used to treat *jaundice, constipation, piles, anaemia and conjnctivitis.* The roots are *purgative, anthelmintic, carminative, rubefacient and anodyne.* It is mainly used in *abdominal pains, constipation, calculus, general anasarca, piles, helminthic infestation, scabies* and *skin disorders.* The root paste is applied to *painful swellings* and *piles* and leaves give relief to *asthma patients.* The seeds are used to cure *snakebites.*

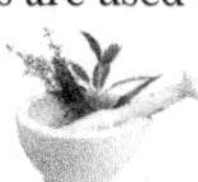

Graceful Sandmat

Botanical Name:
Chamaesyce hypericifolia

Family:
Euphorbiaceae (**Castor family**)

Synonyms:
Chamaesyce glomerifera, Euphorbia glomerifera, Euphorbia hypericifolia

Common Names:
Graceful Sandmat, Graceful spurge, Large spotted spurge, Milk purslane

Description:
Graceful Sandmat is an annual herb with milky sap. Stems are hairless, erect, often red. Oppositely arranged leaves are oblong-elliptic, 1 - 2.5 cm long, 4 - 8 mm wide, margin slightly toothed. The species Name *hypericifolia* means, having leaves like Hypericum, that is, St. John's Wort. Indeed, the leaves do bear a strong resemblance to St Johns Wort's leaves. Flowers are minute, clustered into cup-like cyathia (A cythium is a flower-like object which is not the actual flower). Cyathia borne solitary in the leaf axil and in dense, nearly leafless glomerules constituting lateral branches. Cyathial appendages are petal-like, 4, white to pink, each with a minute gland at the base. Capsules are smooth, generally widest below the middle. Flowering: July-December.

Medicinal Uses:
All parts of the plant are used as *medicine* for *inducing lactation*.

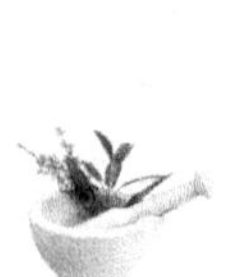

Suryavarti

Botanical Name:

Chrozophora rottleri

Family:

Euphorbiaceae (**Castor family**)

Synonyms:

Croton rottleri

Common Names:

Suryavarti, Rottler's Chrozophora • Hindi: *Shadevi* • Marathi: *Suryavarti* • Tamil: *Purapirakkai* • Telugu: *Erra miriyamu, Guruguchettu, Linga mirapa* • Kannada: *Lingamenasu* • Konkani: *Survarli* • Urdu: *Chotaki hunkatath, Suryawarta* • Sanskrit: *Suryavarta*

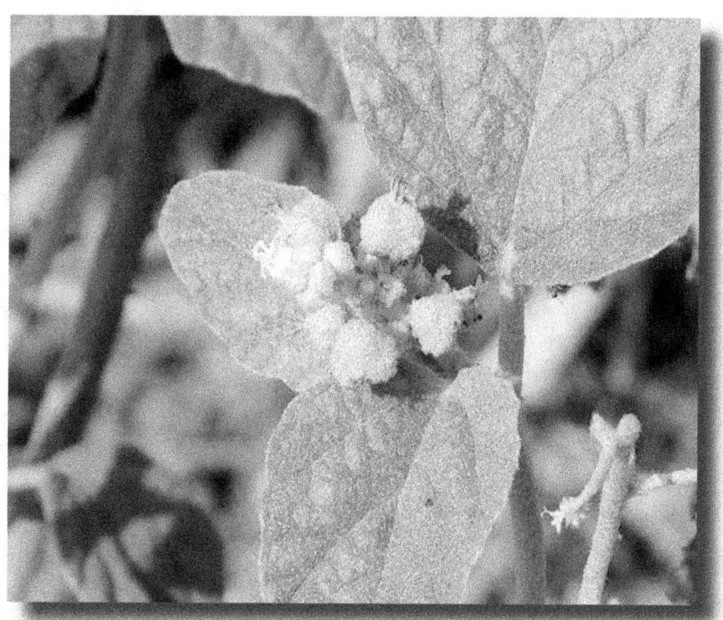

Description:

Suryavarti is an erect herb with silvery hairs. The lower part of the stem is naked, upper part hairy. It has slender tap-root. Leaves are stalked, 3.5-9.5 cm long, 2.3-8 cm wide, ovate to circular, with wavy margin. The leaves are densely hairy on both sides. Flowers are small, yellowish. Male flowers petals ovate. Female flowers sepals triangular, acute. Fruit is a capsule. Flowering: February-August.

Medicinal Uses:

In Nepal, the juice of the fruit is given in cases of *cough* and *cold.*

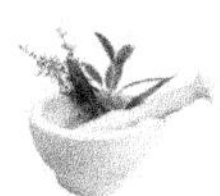

Triangular Spurge

Botanical Name:

Euphorbia antiquorum

Family:

Euphorbiaceae (**Castor family**)

Common Names:

Triangular Spurge, Square Spurge, Square milk hedge, Fleshy spurge • Hindi: _Tridhara, Vajrakantaka_ • Manipuri: _Tengnou_ • Marathi: _Narasya_ • Tamil: _Chaturakalli, Kalli, Kantiravam, Kodiravam, Tiruvargalli_ • Malayalam: _Chaturakkalli_ • Telugu: _Bommajemudu, Bontha jemudu, Bontha kl_ • Kannada: _Kontekalli, Jadekalli, Mundukalli_ • Bengali: _Tiktasij_ • Konkani: _Tirikon_ • Sanskrit: _Snuhu, Vajrakantaka_

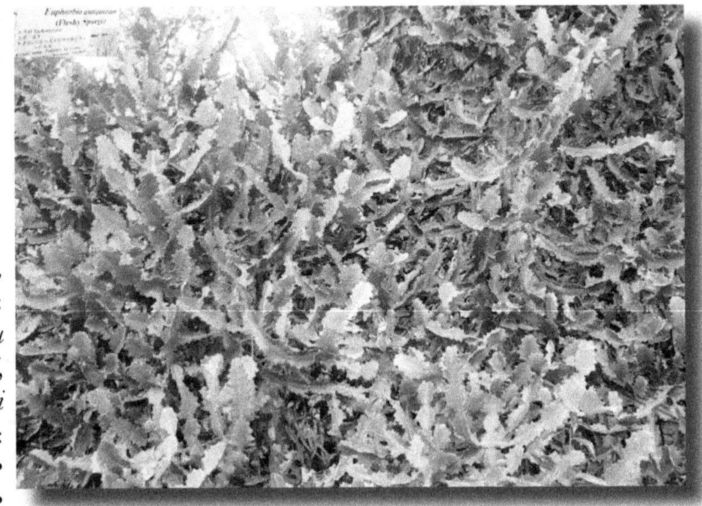

Description:

Triangular Spurge is a small succulent tree, usually shrub-like, with plentiful white sap. Wide spread throughout peninsular India, it can be found growing up to an altitude of 800 m. One of the largest armed tree Euphorbias with an average height of 5-7 m, it has been known to attain gigantic proportions if left undisturbed. Older stems cylindrical, with brownish bark; younger branches smooth, green, distinctly 3(-4)-angled, distinctly articulate with the segments 6-30 by 2-5 cm, drying greenish, with shallow to hardly narrowed sinuses between the spine-shields. Spine-shields in rows, shallow, 1.5-2 cm apart, spines in pairs, (3-)4-6 mm long, blackish, persistent. The flower structures are called cyathia. Cyathium is an inflorescence consisting of a cuplike cluster of modified leaves enclosing a female flower and several male flowers. Yellow cyathia can be in triads or 3-4 individual together. They are full of honey that attract bees. Seed capsules turn deep red on maturity. The odour of its latex is pungent and lingering. Easily propagated from seed or vegetatively, this Euphorbia is common in collections and easy to grow.

Medicinal Uses:

The juice of the plant is useful in _chest pain_ and _constipation_. The latex is applied to boils for _early suppuration_ and _healing_. The root bark is _purgative_ and the latex is useful in killing _maggots of wounds_. The _saline extract_ of the plant is _antibiotic_.

Asthma Weed

Botanical Name:

Euphorbia hirta

Family:

Euphorbiaceae (**Castor family**)

Common Names:

Asthma Weed, Common spurge, Cats hair
• Hindi: *Bara dudhi* • Manipuri: *Pakhamba maton* • Marathi: *Dudhi* • Tamil: *Ammam Paccharisi* • Malayalam: *Nelapalai* • Telugu: *Nanabalu* • Kannada: *Achchedida* • Bengali: *Barokarni* • Konkani: *Dudurli*

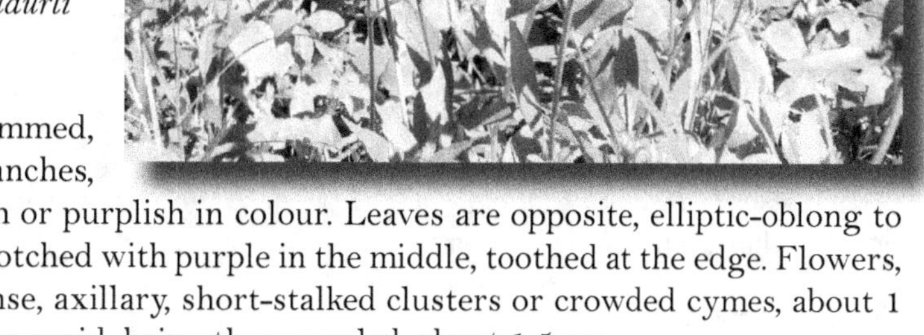

Description:

Asthma Weed is a slender-stemmed, annual hairy plant with many branches, growing up to 40 cms tall, reddish or purplish in colour. Leaves are opposite, elliptic-oblong to oblong-lancelike, 1-2.5 cm long, blotched with purple in the middle, toothed at the edge. Flowers, purplish to greenish in colour, dense, axillary, short-stalked clusters or crowded cymes, about 1 mm in length. Capsules are broadly ovoid, hairy, three-angled, about 1.5 cm.

Medicinal Uses:

The Asthma Weed has traditionally been used in *Asia* to *treat bronchitic asthma* and *laryngeal spasm*, though in modern herbalism, it, is more used in the *treatment of intestinal amoebic dysentery*. It should not be used without *expert's guidance*, since large doses cause *gastro-intestinal irritation*, *nausea* and *vomiting*.

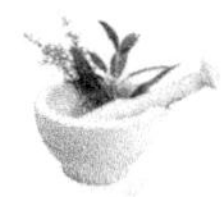

Willow-Leaved Water Croton

Botanical Name:
Homonoia riparia

Family:
Euphorbiaceae (**Castor family**)

Synonyms:
Adelia neriifolia

Common Names:
Willow-Leaved Water Croton
• Hindi: *Sherni* • Marathi: *Raan kaner, Sherni* • Tamil: *Kattalari* • Malayalam: *Neervanchi, Puzhavanchi* • Telugu: *Adavi ganneru* • Kannada: *Hole nage, Niru kanigalu* • Oriya: *Thotthori* • Assamese: *Hil-kadam, Tuipui-sulhla* • Khasi: *Jalangmynrei* • Sanskrit: *Jalavetasa, Kshudrapashanabheda*

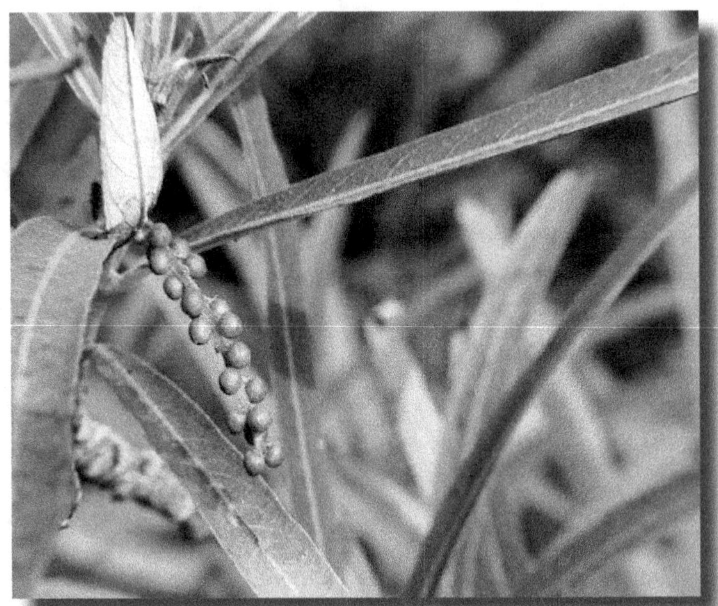

Description:
Willow-Leaved Water Croton is a plant commonly found growing along small streams at low and medium altitudes, on banks, and in streambeds. It is a shrub growing to 1-3 m tall. The leaves are linear-lanceshaped, 12-20 cm long, and 1.5-2 cm wide. Upper surface of the leaves is green and shining, and the lower surface brown and hairy. Reddish flowers are born in spikes 5-10 cm long, with obovate bracts, 1.5-2 mm long. Male flowers have 0.2 mm long stalks, 3 velvety sepals, 3-4 mm long. Female flowers have 5 oblong sepals, with tapering tips, about 1-2 mm long. The capsules are about 8 mm in diameter, hairy, and borne on solitary, hairy spikes, 5-12 cm long, in leaf axils.

Medicinal Uses:
A decoction of the root is a *laxative* and *diuretic*, and is used in *piles, stones in the bladder, gonorrhoea, syphilis* and *thirst*.

Bellyache Bush

Botanical Name:

Jatropha gossypiifolia

Family:

Euphorbiaceae **(Castor family)**

Common Names:

Bellyache Bush, Cotton-leaf physic nut • Hindi: *Ratanjoti* • Manipuri: *E-hidak* • Tamil: *Siria Amanakku* • Malayalam: *Chuvanna Kadalavanakku* • Kannada: *Chikka kada haralu* • Bengali: *Lal bherenda*

Description:

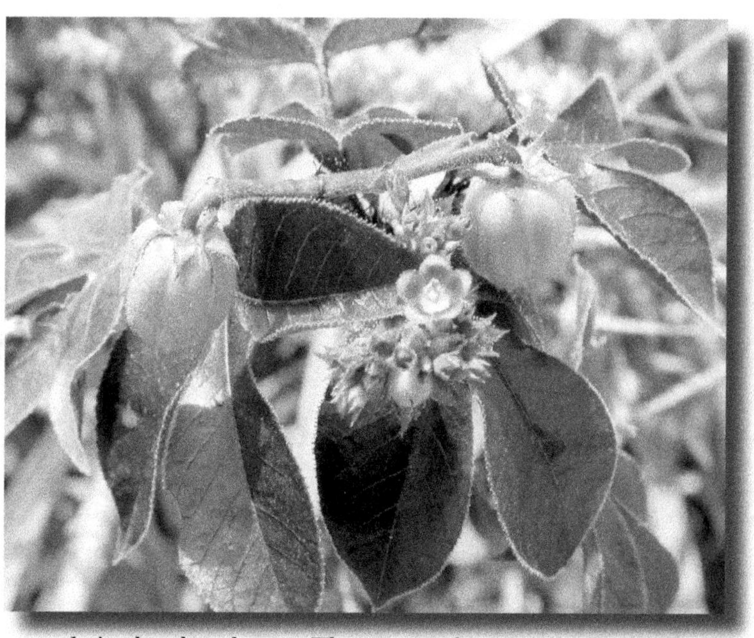

This is a container grown plant but lives outdoors. It is often confused with castor oil plant (Ricinus communis) It grows spontaneously in abandoned areas. The contrast between the purple leaves and green fruits is something special. This bush has beautiful foilage The new leaves on the top of each branch are tri-lobed and a lovely purple-red. Castor oil leaves are larger and with many more labes. The flowers are small, red with yellow centers, and are in small clusters throughout the upper part of the plant. Seed pods are smooth and oval, about the size of a cherry, 12 mm across and contain three to four seeds about 8 mm long. The leaves shine in the sun and it will reach 3' tall and easily as wide in one growing season. The leaves are a glossy, burgundy-red that ages to a medium green. The plant takes the heat and has tremendous vigor. It easily seeds itself around, and can become a weed. The fruits of the plant are poisonous to humans and animals. The toxic substance is a toxalbumin which, when eaten, leads to symptoms of gastro-enteritis and eventual death of some animals.

Medicinal Uses:

It may come as a surprise then to discover that *concoctions* derived from *bellyache bush* are actually used in *folk medicine* all around the world, in particular to treat *bellyache*, and hence, the name, *bellyache bush*. It's a case of "what does not kill us makes us stronger."

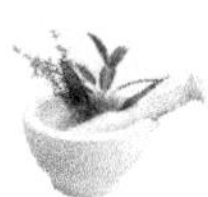

Kamala Tree

Botanical Name:

Mallotus philippensis

Family:

Euphorbiaceae (**Castor family**)

Common Names:

Kamala Tree, Dyer's rottlera, Monkey face tree, Orange kamala, Red kamala, Scarlet croton • Hindi: *Kamala, Raini, Rohan, Rohini, Sinduri* • Manipuri: *Ureirom laba* • Marathi: *Kesari, Shendri* • Tamil: *Kapila poti, Kuranku-mañcanari* • Malayalam: *Cenkolli, Kunkumappuumaram, Kurangumanjas, Naavatta, Nuurimaram* • Telugu: *Kunkuma-chettu* • Kannada: *Kunkuma-damara* • Bengali: *Kamala* • Sanskrit: *Kampilyaka*

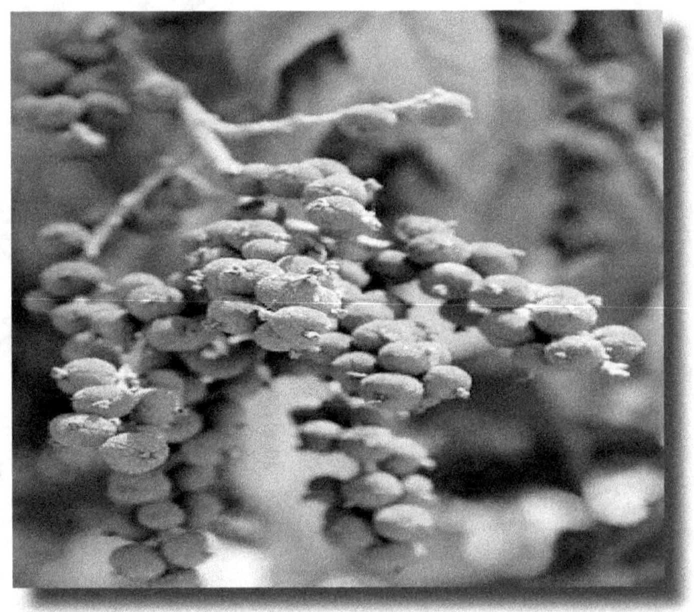

Description:

The Kamala Tree (pronounced *kaamlaa*) is a tree found throughout India. It has been in use as medicinal tree in India for ages. The tree can grow up to 10 m tall. Alternately arranged, ovate or rhombic ovate leaves are rusty-velvety. Male and female flowers occur in different trees. Female flowers are borne in lax spike like racemes at the end of branches or in leaf axils. Male flowers occur three together in the axils of small bracts. Capsule is trigonous-globular, covered with a bright crimson layer of minute, easily detachable reddish powder. Kamala is supposed to be a very useful tree. It is source of Kamala dye which is used in colouring silk and wool. It is used as anti-oxidant for ghee and vegetable oils. Oil is used as hair-fixer and added in ointment. Seed oil is used in paints and varnishes. Seed cake is used as manure.

Medicinal Uses:

According to *Ayurveda*, *leaves* are *bitter*, *cooling* and an *appetizer*. The fruit, when heated is used as a *purgative*, *anthelmintic*, *vulnerary*, *detergent*, *maturant*, *carminative*, *alexiteric* and useful in the treatment of *bronchitis*, *abdominal diseases*, *spleen enlargement*, etc.

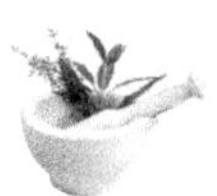

Castor Bean Plant

Botanical Name:

Ricinus communis

Family:

Euphorbiaceae (**Castor family**)

Common Names:

Castor bean, Castor oil plant, Wonder tree • Hindi: *Arandi* • Manipuri: *Kege* • Tamil: *Amanakku, Vilakkennai Kottaimuttu* • Kannada: *Oudla* • Bengali: *Veranda* • Assamese: *Era-gach* • Malayalam: *Chittamankku*

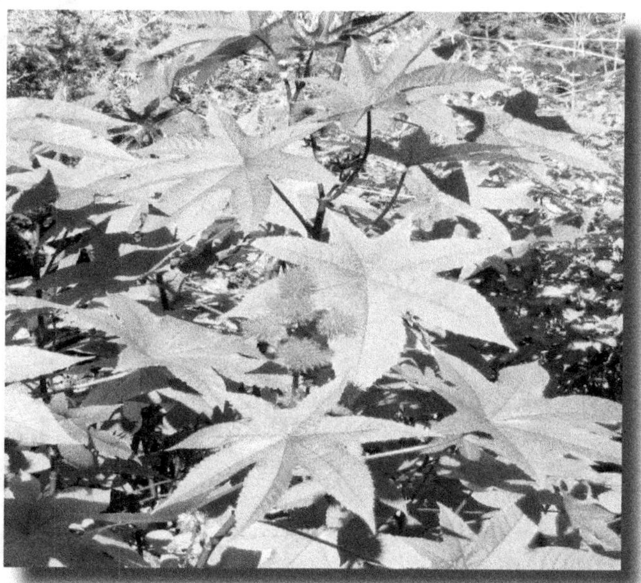

Description:

The castor bean plant, an erect, tropical shrub or small tree, grows up to 30 feet tall. As an annual in the cooler zones, it grows up to 15' tall. It is a very fast growing plant. The joints of the hollow stem, stalks and leaves are reddish to purple. The 6 - 11 lobed, palmate leaves with uneven serrated edge, are also red or coloured and often have a blue-gray bloom. There is also a green variety. The flat seeds are in a seedpod that explodes when ripen. All the top of the stem and stalks are the inflorescence with the male - and female flowers. The female flowers are the fuzzy red structures at the top of the flower spike with the male flowers positioned on the lower half, and have conspicuous yellow anthers. The oblong fruit turns brown when ripe. In each seed pod (a capsule) there are three seeds. The seeds of castor bean or castor oil plant, are very poisonous to people, animals and insects; just one milligram of ricin (one of the main toxic proteins in the plant) can kill an adult. The castor oil is extracted from the beans, which is used for medicinal purposes. Commercially prepared castor oil contains none of the toxin.

Medicinal Uses:

In Manipur, the leaves of this plant are warmed, crushed and applied to the *anus* as a remedy for *bleeding piles*. The seed oil is used as a purgative. The leaf-paste is used as *poultice* on *sores, gouts* or *rheumatic swellings*. The decoction of the roots is given in *lumbago*. For lactation, leaves of the plant are heated and applied to a *woman's breasts* to *improve the secretion of milk, particularly after childbirth.*

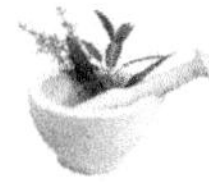

Red Sandalwood

Botanical Name:
Adenanthera pavonina

Family:
Fabaceae (**Pea family**)

Synonyms:
Adenanthera gersenii, Adenanthera polita, Corallaria parvifolia

Common Names:
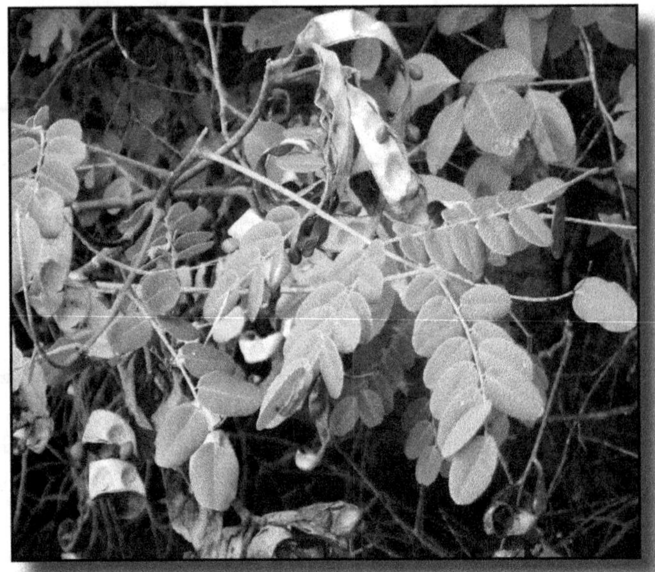

Red Sandalwood, Coral-wood, Peacock flower fence, Red beadtree • Hindi: *Rakt chandan, Badi gumchi* • Marathi: *Thorla goonj* • Tamil: *Ani kundamani, Manjadi* • Malayalam: *Sem, Manchadi* • Telugu: *Gurivenda, Enugaguruginji* • Kannada: *Ane golaganji* • Bengali: *Ranjana* • Oriya: *Sokakainjo* • Konkani: *Odlygunji* • Assamese: *Chandan* • Gujarati: *Badigumchi* • Sanskrit: *Ksharaka, kunchandana, Tamraka*

Description:
Red Sandalwood is a timber tree. This plant is found in the wild in India. Leaves are compound bipinnate, green when young, turning yellow when old. The small, yellowish flower grows in dense drooping rat-tail flower heads, almost like cat-tail flower-heads. Fruits are curved, hanging, green pods that turn brown, coil up and split open as they ripen to reveal small bright red seeds. These attractive seeds have been used as beads in jewellery, leis and rosaries. They were also used in ancient India for weighing gold. The seeds are curiously similar in weight. Four seeds make up about one gramme. Children love the hard red seeds and few can resist collecting the brightly coloured seeds usually littered under the tree. The young leaves can be cooked and eaten. the wood is extremely hard and used in boat-building and making furniture.

Medicinal Uses:
A red powder made from the wood is also used as an *antiseptic paste*. In *Ancient Indian medicine*, the *grounded seeds* are used to treat *boils and inflammations*. A decoction of the leaves is used to treat *gouts* and *rheumatism*. The bark is used to *wash hair.*

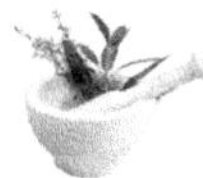

Red Bush Tea

Botanical Name:

Aspalathus linearis

Family:

Fabaceae (**Pea family**)

Common Names:

Red Bush Tea, Rooibos Tea, South African red tea

Description:

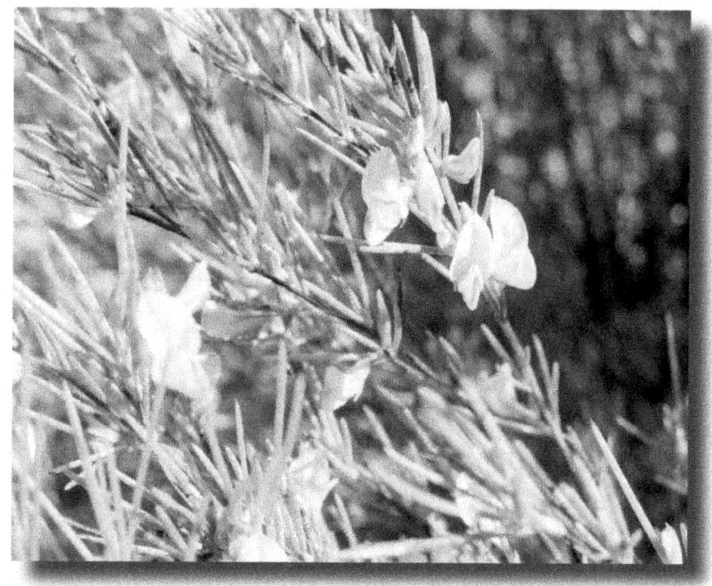

Rooibos or Red Bush Tea is a shrub which can grow up to 2 meter in height. The erects red coloured rooibos stems contain many dark green needle shaped leaves. The rooibos shrub produces small yellow flowers in spring through early summer. Each flower produces a one seeded small bean. Roobos has a long tap root, sometimes up to 2 m in length, enabling the plant to survive periods of drought. Rooibos grows only in South Africa. Rooibos tea is much appreciated because it does not contain caffeine and is low in tannins. The seed have been recently brought to South India also by some plant lovers.

Medicinal Uses:

Rooibos has *anti-carcinogenic* and *antimutagenic* effects. Tea made with it is used for its *anti-inflammatory* and *anti-allergic properties.* The consumption of Rooibos Tea may *relief fever, asthma, insomnia, colic in infants* and *skin disorders.*The Rooibos extracts are used in *ointments against eczema.*

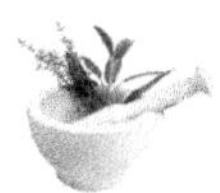

Himalayan Milk Vetch

Botanical Name:
Astragalus floridus

Family:
Fabaceae (**Pea family**)

Common Names:
Himalayan milk vetch, Milk vetch

Description:
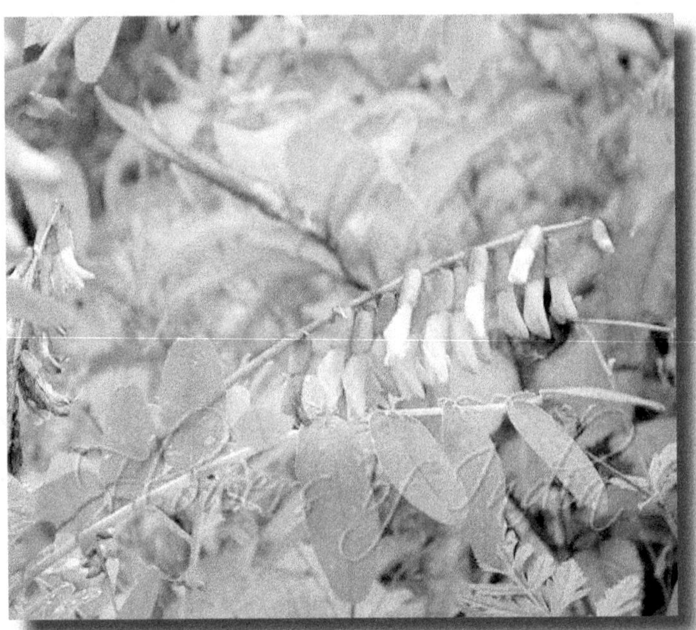

Himalayan Milk Vetch is a member of the *pea family,* includes many species that grow around the world. Himalayan Milk Vetch is an herbaceous perennial native to the Himalayas. The multi-stemmed plant grows to about 1 to 1.5 m in height and has alternate, compound leaves composed of 12 to 18 pairs of small leaflets. Mature plants have yellow pea-like flowers in long clusters during early summer. These are followed by seedpods growing up to 15 cm in length. The roots are rhizomatous, black with a yellow core, have a peculiar odour and a sweetish taste.

Medicinal Uses:
Astragalus has recently come into prominence in the *United States* for its *medicinal properties,* but it has long been known in *traditional Chinese medicine* to invigorate vital *energy and strengthen resistance to diseases.* There, the dried roots are frequently sold and are boiled along with other herbs or even chicken broth to prepare *a tonic or medicinal soup.* The roots are used for its *immunostimulant, antimicrobial, cardiotonic* and *diuretic* properties. Because it increases the production of *white blood cells,* it has been found useful in *therapy for cancer patients* that have undergone *chemotherapy* or *radiation.* It has also been used *for treating chronic diarrhoea* and *reducing blood pressure,* and for *treating common colds.* Astragalus has been marketed as *dried roots, ground roots* in *tablets* and *capsule form, liquid extracts,* or as a *component in herbal tea.*

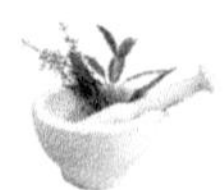

Takoli

Botanical Name:
Dalbergia lanceolaria ssp. lanceolaria

Family:
Fabaceae (**Pea family**)

Common Names:
Takoli • Hindi: *Takoli* • Telugu: *Nagulapachari* • Assamese: *Meda-luwa* • Malayalam: *Mannavitti* • Tamil: *Erigai* • Marathi: *Dandus* • Oriya: *Dodilo* • Rajasthani: *parbati* • Urdu: *Dandous*

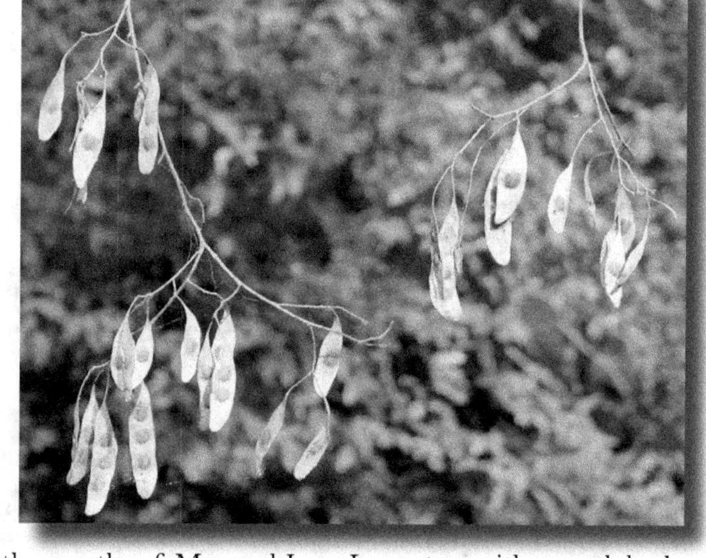

Description:
Takoli is a very conspicuous and handsome tree when flowering, which appear very profusely during the months of May and June. Large tree with smooth bark, branches glabrous. Leaf compound 7.0-15.0 cm long; leaflets 11-17, 2.5-5.0 cm long, ovate or obovate or elliptic, often emarginate, glabrous, glaucous. Inflorescence large axillary or terminal panicles flowers unilaterally arranged. Calyx silky pubescent, upper teeth obtuse, lower 3 longer and acute. Flower tube dull white or pinkish. Vexillum c. 5-10 mm long. Stamens 10, in 2 groups of 5 stamens each. Fruit c. 5-8 cm long, narrowed at both ends, glabrous, usually 1-seeded.

Medicinal Uses:
The sweet blackish pulp of the seedpod is used as a *mild laxative*.

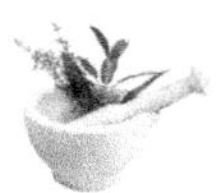

Shisham

Botanical Name:

Dalbergia sissoo

Family:

Fabaceae (**Pea family**)

Common Names:

Indian rosewood Hindi: *Shisham* • Manipuri: *Sissu* • Bengali: *Sitral*

Description:

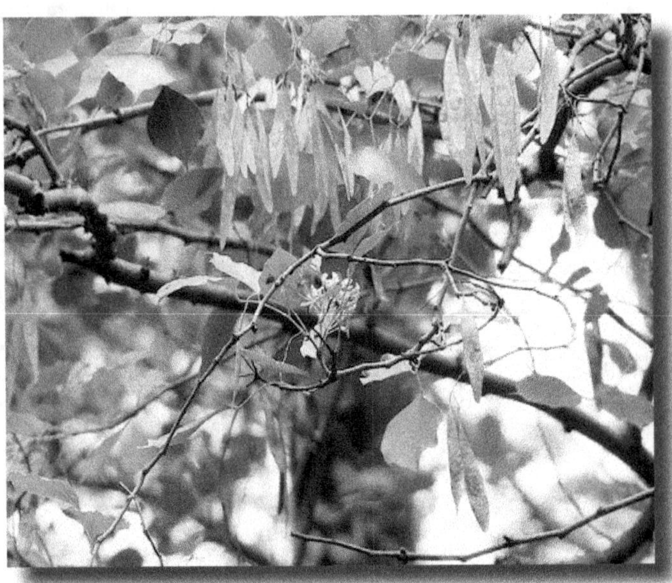

Shisham is a medium to a large deciduous tree, native to India, with a light crown which reproduces by seeds and suckers. It can grow up to a maximum of 25 m in height and 2 to 3 m in diameter, but is usually smaller. Trunks are often crooked when grown in the open. Leaves are leathery, alternate, pinnately compound and about 15 cm long. Flowers are whitish to pink, fragrant, nearly sessile, up to 1.5 cm long and in dense clusters 5-10 cm in length. Pods are oblong, flat, thin, strap-like 4-8 cm long, 1 cm wide, and light brown. They contain 1-5 flat bean-shaped seeds 8-10 mm long. They have a long taproot and numerous surface roots which produce suckers. It is primarily found growing along river banks below 900 m elevation, but can range naturally up to 1300 m. Shisham is best known internationally as a premier timber species of the rosewood genus. However, Shisham is also an important fuel wood, shade, and shelter. With its multiple products, tolerance of light frosts and long dry seasons, this species deserves greater consideration for tree farming, reforestation and agro forestry applications. After teak, it is the most important cultivated timber tree in India, planted on roadsides, and as a shade tree for tea plantations.

Medicinal Uses:

The decoction of leaves is useful in *gonorrhoea*. The root is an astringent and the Wood is an alternative, useful in l*eprosy, boils, eruptions* and to *allay vomiting*.

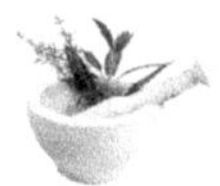

West Indian Indigo

Botanical Name:

Indigofera suffruticosa

Family:

Fabaceae (**Pea family**)

Synonyms:

Indigofera anil

Common Names:

West Indian Indigo, Anil, Small-leaved indigo, Guatemalan indigo, Wild indigo • Hindi: *Vilayati nil* • Marathi: *Nilambi* • Tamil: *Chimai-nili* • Sanskrit: *Nilika, Nilini, Vishashodhani*

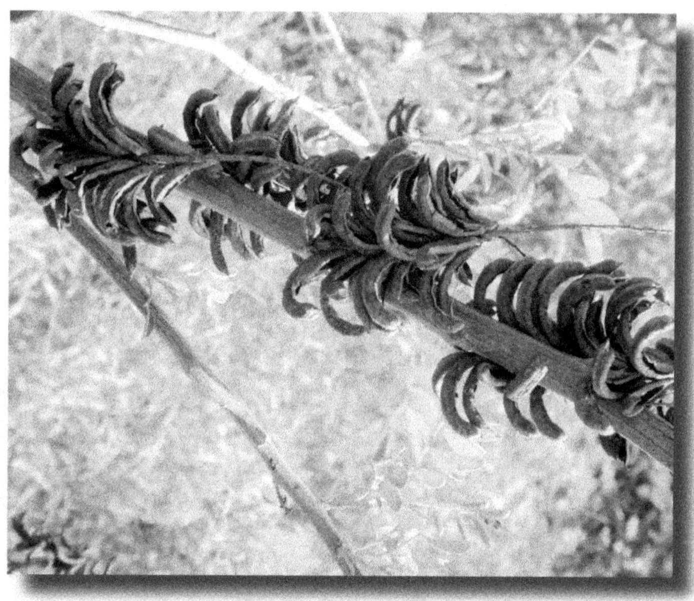

Description:

The West Indian Indigo is an erect, branched, half-woody shrub, growing to a height of about one metre. The stems are sparsely covered with short hairs. The leaves are 5-8 cm long. The leaflets are 9-11, oblong to oblong-elliptic, 1-2 cm long, pale, and hairy beneath. The flowers are red, about 5 mm long, and borne on axillary and solitary racemes 2-3 cm long. The pods are numerous, crowded, reflexed, strongly curved, and 1-1.5 cm long, and contain 6-8 seeds. This species is one of the sources of natural indigo, and along with Indigifolera tinctoria, represents the chief commercial indigo. It is cultivated as green manure in Malaya and Java. It is used as a perennial cover crop for coffee. West Indian Indigo is a native of Tropical America, but widely naturalized in India.

Medicinal Uses:

In Brazil, the West Indian Indigo is one of the *reputed remedies for snakebites,* and in the United States, it is often applied to the *stings of bees* and other *insects.* In Mexico, the *leaves as a cataplasm or in decoction* are applied to the *forehead of children with fever* and to any *painful area.* The *seeds in powder form* are a cure for *ulcers.*

Pongam Tree

Botanical Name:

Millettia pinnata

Family:

Fabaceae (**Pea family**)

Synonyms:

Pongamia pinnata, Pongamia glabra, Derris indica, Cytisus pinnatus

Common Names:

Pongam Tree, Indian Beech Tree, Pongame Oil Tree • Hindi: *Karanj* • Tamil: *Punnai* • Malayalam: *Ponnu, Unnu* • Oriya: *Koranjo* • Kannada: *Honge* • Marathi: *Karanj* • Telugu: *Pungu* • Gujarati: *Karanja* • Bengali: *Karanj* • Assamese: *Karchaw* • Sanskrit: *Karanjah*

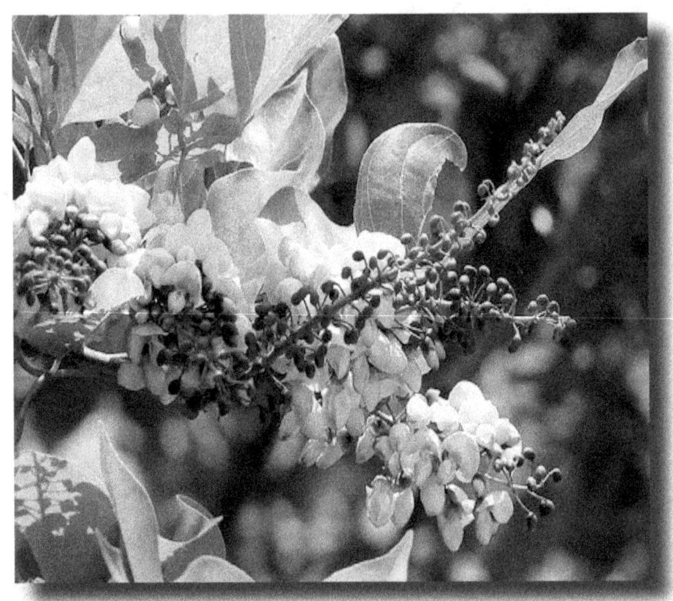

Description:

A fast-growing deciduous tree up to 20 meters tall that is thought to have originated in India and is found throughout Asia. It is a deciduous tree that grows to about 15-25 meters in height with a large canopy that spreads equally wide. The leaves are a soft, shiny burgundy in early summer and mature to a glossy, deep green as the season progresses. Small clusters of white, purple, and pink flowers blossom on their branches throughout the year, maturing into brown seed pods. The tree is well suited to intense heat and sunlight and its dense network of lateral roots and its thick, long taproot make it drought tolerant. Flowering: March-April.

Medicinal Uses:

A thick brownish oil can be extracted from the *large seeds*, and is used *industrially in medicines*, notably for the treatment of *rheumatism*.

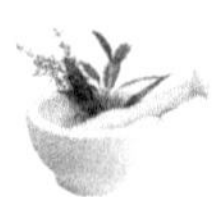

Velvet Bean

Botanical Name:

Mucuna pruriens

Family:

Fabaceae (**Bean family**)

Common Names:

Velvet bean, Cowitch, Cowhage, Kapikachu, Nescafe, Sea bean • Hindi: *Kiwach* • Marathi: *Khaj-kuiri* • Malayalam: *Naicorna* • Telugu: *Pilliadugu* • Kannada: *Nayisonanguballi* • Bengali: *Akolchi* • Tamil: *Punaippidukkan*

Description:

The Velvet Bean is an annual, climbing shrub with long vines that can reach over 15 metres. Leaves are trifoliate, gray-silky beneath; petioles are long and silky, and 6-11 cm. Leaflets are membranous, terminal leaflets are smaller, lateral very unequal sided. Dark purple flowers (6 to 30) occur in drooping racemes. Fruits are curved, 4-6 seeded. The longitudinally ribbed pod, is densely covered with loose orange hairs which cause a severe itch if they come in contact with the skin. The beans are shiny black or brown. It is found in tropical Africa, India and the Caribbean.

Medicinal Uses:

The Velvet Bean can be beneficial, since it is high in levodopa which helps *maintain healthy cholesterol* and *blood sugar levels.* The seed powder of *Mucuna pruriens* has long been used in *Ayurvedic medicine* for diseases including *parkinsonism,* and has proven in medical tests to have equal or superior effectiveness in the treatment of *parkinsons disease* over *conventional, synthetic levodopa* medications. Another benefit of *Mucuna* is that it can increase the production of human growth hormone, and extracts are commonly sold as *body-building supplements.*

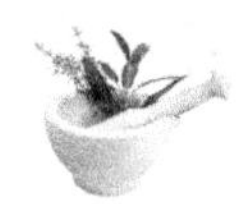

Tree Bean

Botanical Name:

Parkia timoriana

Family:

Fabaceae (**Pea family**)

Synonyms:

Parkia javanica, Parkia roxburghii

Common Names:

Tree Bean • Hindi: *Sapota, Khorial* • Manipuri: *Yongchak* • Kannada: *Shivalingada mara* • Marathi: *Unkampinching* • Assamese: *Khorial*

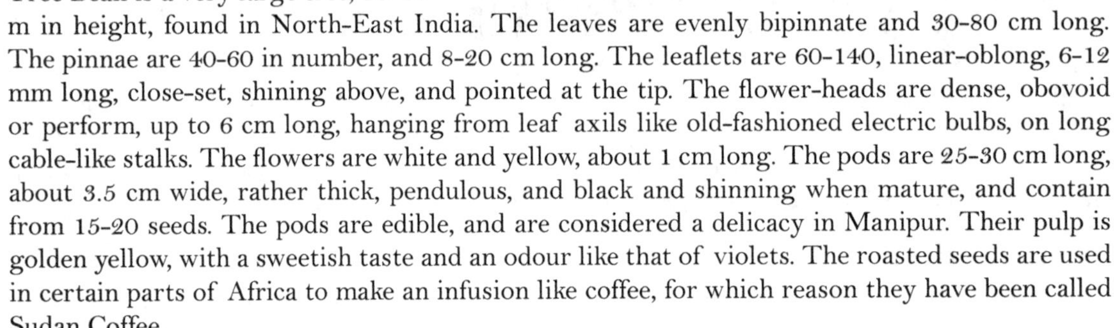

Description:

Tree Bean is a very large tree, 25-40 m in height, found in North-East India. The leaves are evenly bipinnate and 30-80 cm long. The pinnae are 40-60 in number, and 8-20 cm long. The leaflets are 60-140, linear-oblong, 6-12 mm long, close-set, shining above, and pointed at the tip. The flower-heads are dense, obovoid or perform, up to 6 cm long, hanging from leaf axils like old-fashioned electric bulbs, on long cable-like stalks. The flowers are white and yellow, about 1 cm long. The pods are 25-30 cm long, about 3.5 cm wide, rather thick, pendulous, and black and shinning when mature, and contain from 15-20 seeds. The pods are edible, and are considered a delicacy in Manipur. Their pulp is golden yellow, with a sweetish taste and an odour like that of violets. The roasted seeds are used in certain parts of Africa to make an infusion like coffee, for which reason they have been called Sudan Coffee.

Medicinal Uses:

Pods are used in *bleeding piles*. The *bark extract* is given in *diarrhoea* and *dysentery*. The *bark and leaves* are employed for making *lotion* and are applied to *sores* and *skin infections*.

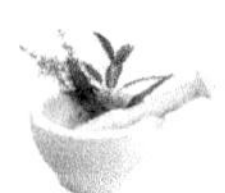

Salaparni

Botanical Name:

Pseudarthria viscida

Family:

Fabaceae (**Pea family**)

Synonyms:

Hedysarum viscidum

Common Names:

Salaparni • Hindi: *Chapakno* • Tamil: *Nirmalli* • Malayalam: *Muvvila, Moovila* • Telugu: *Nayakuponna, Muyyakuponna* • Sanskrit: *Salaparni, Sanaparni*

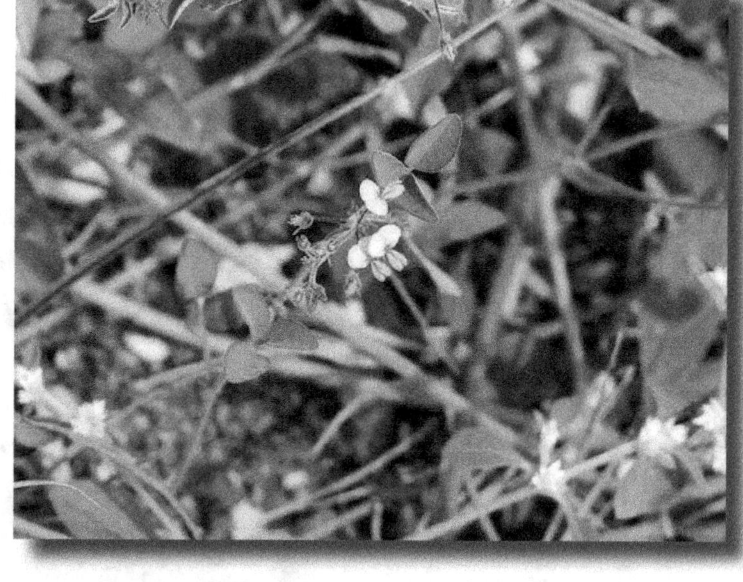

Description:

Salaparni is a perennial under shrub which grows all over India up to 1000 m altitude. It attains the height about 60-120 cm. The branches are slender and covered with minute white hair. The leaves are 7.5-15 cm long and 2.5-5 cm broad, trifoliate, ovate-oblong, hairy and densely grey-silky beneath. The flowers purplish or pink, in 15-30 cm long axillary racemes. The fruits, pods, oblong, flattened, covered with sticky hairs. The seeds 4-6, compressed and brownish black in colour. The plant flowers in May.

Medicinal Uses:

The whole plant of Salaparni is used for *medicinal purpose* in *Ayurvedic medicine.* The herb is seldom used externally. Internally, it is useful in vast range of diseases. It is used in the *treatment of asthma* and *nervous dysfunction.* It is also used in the treatment of *insect bites* and used against *inflammations, vomiting,* etc.

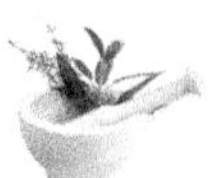

Indian Kudzu

Botanical Name:
Pueraria tuberosa

Family:
Fabaceae (**Pea family**)

Common Names:
Indian kudzu • Hindi: *Sural, Bilaikand, Bharda, Tirra, Bankumra* • Bengali: *Shimia batraji* • Marathi: *Ghorbel* • Gujrati: *Vidarikand* • Telugu: *Darigummadi* • Kannada: *Gumadigida* • Malayalam: *Mutukku* • Sanskrit: *Bhukushmandi*

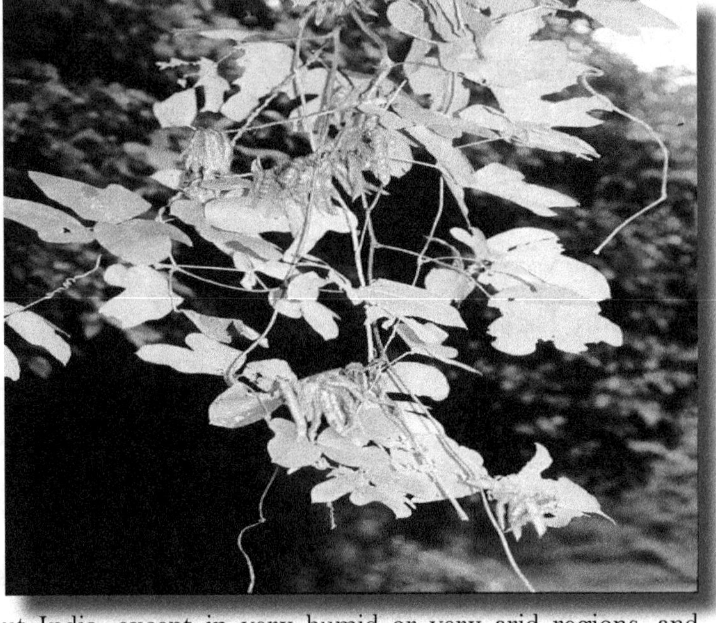

Description:
Indian kudzu is a large perennial climber with very large tuberous roots, distributed nearly throughout India, except in very humid or very arid regions, and ascending up to 1,200 m. Woody stems grow up to 12 cm in diameter. Leaves are divided into 3. Flowers blue or purplish blue, in 15-30 cm long racemes. Pods are flat and 5-7 cm long, densely clothed with long, silky, bristly brown hairs; seeds 3-6.

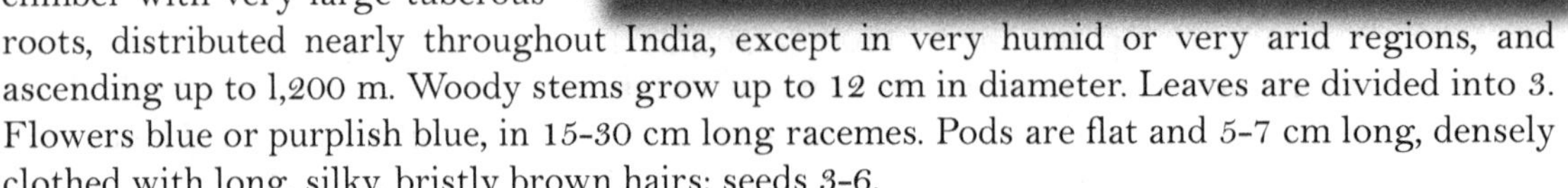

Medicinal Uses:
In *Ayurveda*, this *herb* is used as a *general tonic*, for *headaches*, and as *a aphrodisiac*. The *roots* are said to be used in medicine as a *demulcent* and *refrigent* in *fevers*, as cataplasm for *swelling of joints*, and as *lactagogue*. It is also *emetic*, *galactogogue* and *tonic*. *Now-a-days*, it is used in preparing *sexual potency enhancement pills*.

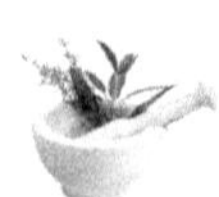

Sensitive Smithia

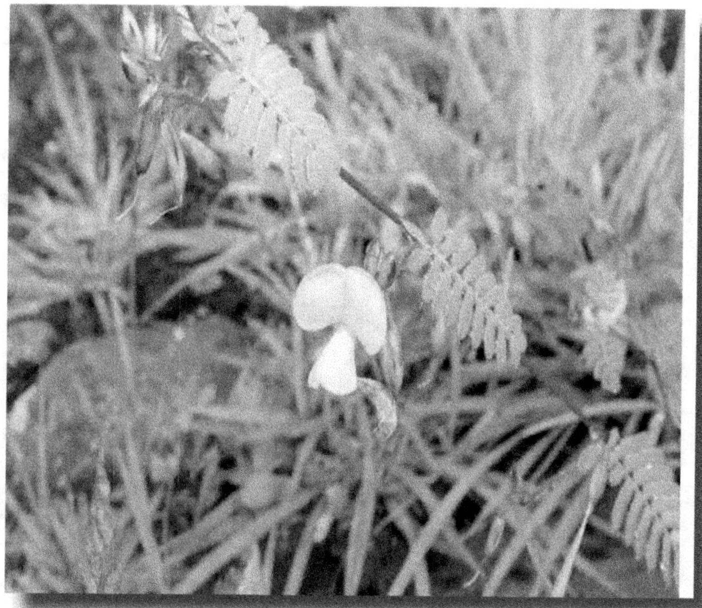

Botanical Name:
Smithia sensitiva

Family:
Fabaceae (**Pea family**)

Common Names:
Sensitive Smithia • Hindi: *Odabirni* • Marathi: *Lajalu kavla* • Bengali: *Nalakashina*

Description:
Sensitive Smithia is a low-growing annual herb, 30-90 cm, common along the roads. It appears at waning of the monsoons. Compound leaves are slightly sensitive to touch. There are 3-10 pairs of oblong leaflets, each 6-12 mm long. Yellow pea-like flowers occur in racemes of 2-6, arising from leaf axils. Flowers are 1.3 cm long. Pods are flat, 1 cm long. Flowers are eaten by the red black spotted blister beetles. Leaves and pods are cooked and eaten. Flowering: August-October.

Medicinal Uses:
The herb is boiled and given as *gravel and for those having difficulty in taking food.* Leaves are *refrigerant* and *stimulate the flow of milk in mothers.* The *juice of the leaves* is used as a *lotion* in *headaches.*

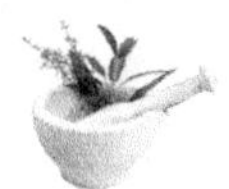

Trefle Gros

Botanical Name:

Tadehagi triquetrum

Family:

Fabaceae **(Pea family)**

Synonyms:

Desmodium triquetrum, Hedysarum triquetrum, Pteroloma triquetrum

Common Names:

Trefle Gros • Malayalam: *Adkhapanal, Chattagai, Kattarali* • Telugu: *Dammidi* • Kannada: *Dodotte, Molada gida* • Assamese: *Ulucha* • Mizo: *Arhrikreh*

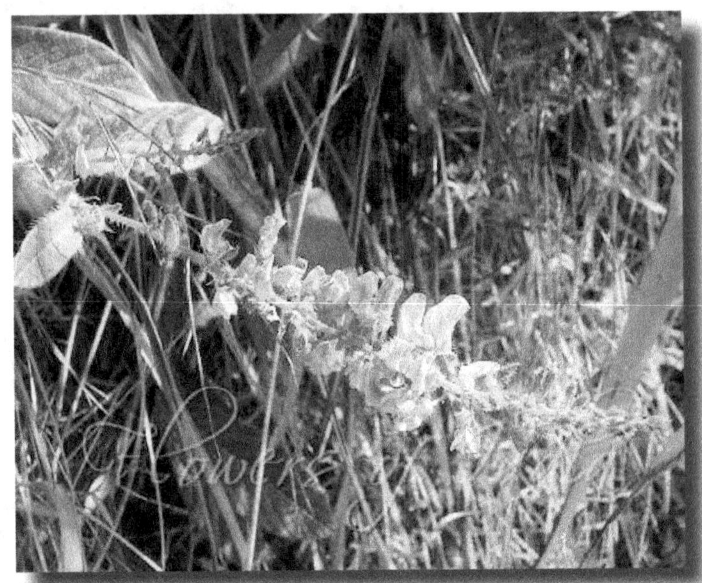

Description:

Trefle Gros is a subshrub, growing up to 3 m tall,t with erect stems which are almost woody. Branches are triangular in cross section, velvety. Leaves are alternately arranged, and the leaf stalk has prominently wings. Leaves are linear-oblong, ovate or heart-shaped, with a tapering tip. Flowers arise in many-flowered racemes in leaf axils. Flowers are small, shaped like pea flowers, pale violet. Legumes are hairy, 5-8 jointed. Flowering: nearly all year.

Medicinal Uses:

Trefle Gros is used to *expel worms, treats spasms in infants, indigestion, piles and abscesses* (whole plant); for *invigorating the spleen* and *promoting digestion* (decoction of whole plant); for hemorrhoids (leaves); for *stomach discomfort* (infusion of leaves); as a *poultice on bruises and drunk daily for chronic coughs* and *tuberculosis* (decoction of roots); to treat *kidney complaints* (infusion of roots); eaten or used in baths for *gastro-intestinal and urinary problems* ranging from an *upset stomach to hepatitis (infusion or decoction of roots).*

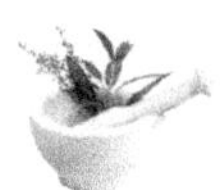

Wild Indigo

Botanical Name:

Tephrosia purpurea

Family:

Fabaceae (**Pea family**)

Common Names:

Wild Indigo, Fish Poison, Tephrosia • Hindi: *Sarphonk, Sharpunkha* • Marathi: *Unhali*

Description:

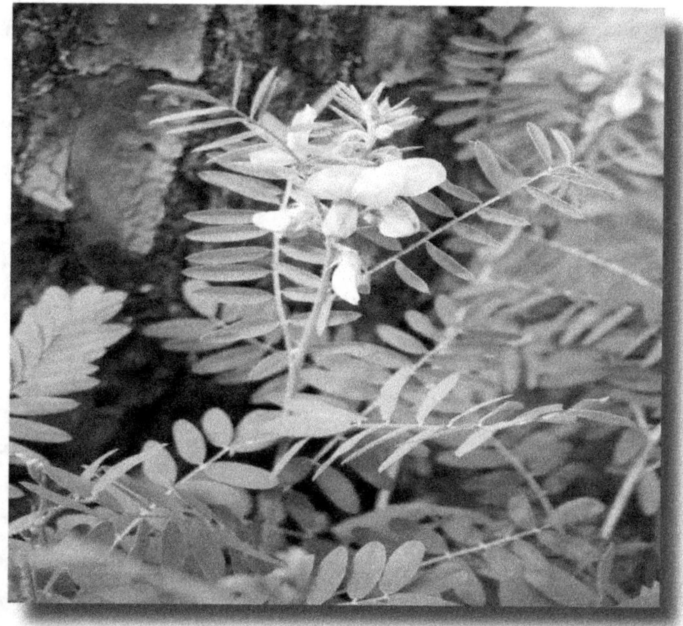

Native to East India, Wild Indigo grows as common wasteland weed. In many parts it is under cultivation as green manure crop. Its is a plant of the genus Tephrosia having pinnate leaves and white or purplish flowers and flat hairy pods. This plant contains a mild toxin called tephrosin which chemically stuns fish but does not effect mammals. The extract is obtained by crushing the whole plant by mortar and pestle, or rocks, and then scattering it in tide pools. In a few minutes, small fish would float up to the surface and could be caught by hand. The flesh from the fish is safe to eat. This system of fishing, good for older people and children, was called hola.

Medicinal Uses:

According to *Ayurveda*, the plant is *digestible, anthelmintic, alexiteric, antipyretic, alternative* and cures diseases of *liver, spleen, heart, blood, tumours, ulcers, leprosy, asthma, poisoning,* etc. According to the Unani system of medicine, the root is *diuretic, allays thirst, enriches blood, cures diarrhoea, useful in bronchitis, asthma, liver, spleen diseases, inflammations, boils and pimples.* Leaves are *tonic to intestines* and a promising *appetiser.* Good for *piles, syphilis* and *gonorrhoea.*

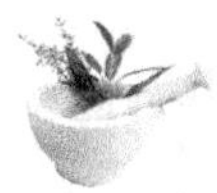

Red Clover

Botanical Name:

Trifolium pratense

Family:

Fabaceae (**Pea family**)

Common Names:

Red Clover, Purple clover, Broad-leaved clover • Hindi: *Tripatra*

Description:

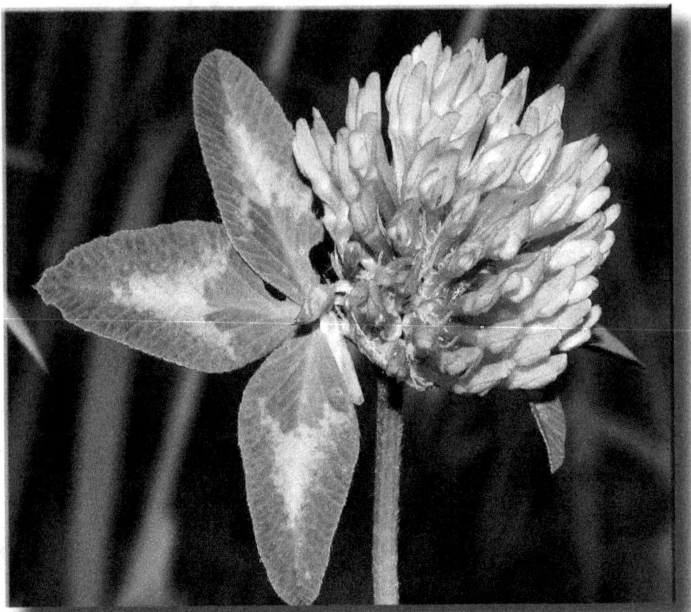

Red Clover is a species of clover, native to Europe, western Asia and northwest Africa. It can be easily distinguished from its close cousin White Clover by its much larger plant, with distinctly pink blooms. It is a herbaceous perennial plant, very variable in size, growing to more than 2 feet tall. The leaves are trifoliate (with three leaflets), each leaflet 15-30 mm long and 8-15 mm broad, green with a characteristic pale crescent in the outer half of the leaf; the petiole is 1-4 cm long, with two basal stipules. The flowers are dark pink with a paler base, 12-15 mm long, produced in a dense inflorescence 2-3 cm diameter. The plant was Named Trifolium pratense by Carolus Linnaeus in 1753. The botanical Name *pratense* is Latin for "found in meadows", which is very much true. It is the national flower of Denmark.

Medicinal Uses:

A *tea from the flower* has long been considered an *antispasmodic* and *mild sedative* and has been used for various *lung and throat problems*, such as *sore throats, cough* and *asthma*. The flowers were once smoked as an *asthma treatment*. Externally, it is used as a *salve for burns* and *sores*. There seems to be no scientific evidence to support medical uses of Clover, but being edible, it probably can't hurt unless it is used instead of more effective treatments.

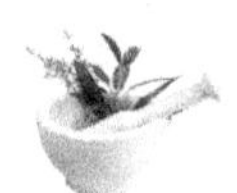

Coffee Plum

Botanical Name:
Flacourtia jangomas

Family:
Flacourtiaceae (**Coffee Plum family**)

Synonyms:
Stigmarota jangomas, Flacourtia cataphrata

Common Names:
Coffee Plum, Indian cherry, Indian plum, Rukam, Runeala plum • Hindi: *Talispatri, Paniala, Pani amla* • Manipuri *Heitroi* • Marathi: *Champeran* • Tamil: *Vaiyyankarai* • Malayalam: *Vayyamkaitha* • Telugu: *Kuragayi* • Kannada: *Chankali, Goraji* • Bengali: *Paniala* • Oriya: *Baincha* • Konkani: *Jagam* • Assamese: *Ponial* • Gujarati: *Talispatra* • Sanskrit: *Sruvavrkash, Vikankatah*

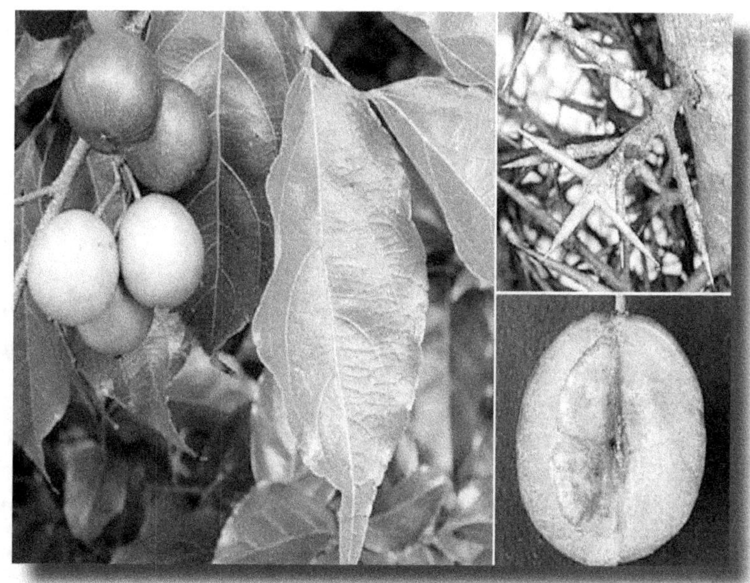

Description:
Coffee Plum is small, deciduous tree, growing to 6-10 m tall. Trunk and branches are commonly thornless in old trees, but densely beset with simple or branched, woody thorns when younger. Bark is light-brown to copper-red or pinkish-buff, flaky. Young branches white-dotted by numerous circular lenticels. Leaves narrow-ovate to ovate-oblong, rarely ovate-lancelike, long-obtuse-acuminate, base broadly wedge-shaped to rounded. Leaves are smooth, shining above, mostly dull beneath, somewhat toothed, 7-10 X 3-4 cm. Leaf stalk is 6-8 mm long. Flowers arise in few flowered clusters in leaf axils. Flowers smell of honey, and looks like small yellowish-white balls of stamens. Male and female flowers are different and are on different trees. Coffee plum is a rounded red to dark purple fruit, that is about an inch wide. It is edible, and is relatively juicy. It can be eaten raw, or transformed into juice or marmalades. Flowering: April-May.

Medicinal Uses:
The *fruits and leaves* are used against *diarrhoea*. Dried leaves are used for *bronchitis* and the roots are used *against toothaches*.

Fried Egg Tree

Botanical Name:
Oncoba spinosa

Family:
Flacourtiaceae

Common Names:
Snuff-box Tree, Fried Egg Tree

Description:
Fried Egg Tree is a spiny shrub or small tree. It grows up to 5 m, but may sometimes reach a height of 8 m. The bark of this plant is mottled grey and rather smooth. The young branches are conspicuously speckled with lenticels (a slightly raised, lens-shaped area on the surface of the

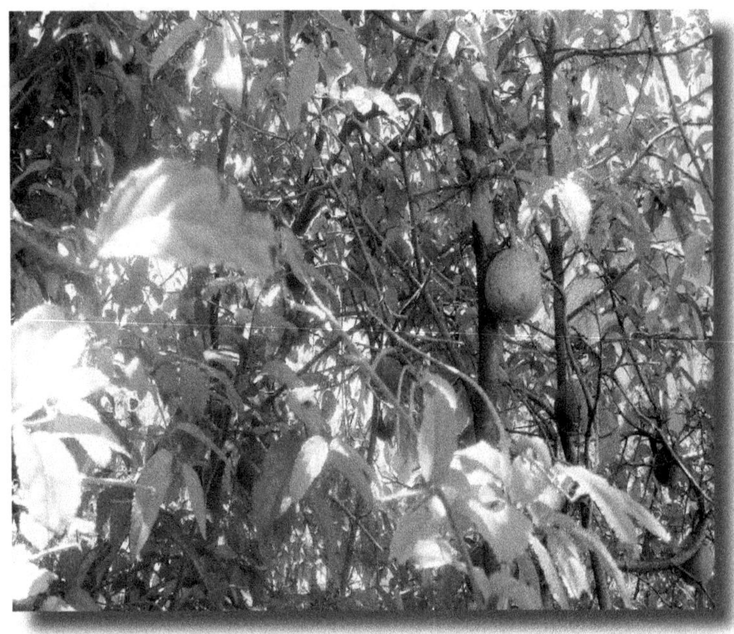

young stems that helps with the exchange of gasses between the plant and the surrounding air). The spines are straight and up to 50 mm in length. The leaves are simple, ovate–elliptic in form with a somewhat pointed tip and rounded, broad base. The leaves are dark, glossy green in colour and somewhat leathery and hairless. The margins are coarsely toothed. The flowers are 3 inch across, white, honey-fragrant and solitary. The fruits have a sour, edible pulp. Beautiful white and yellow flowers look like 'fried eggs' when they drop off and fall on the ground with their yellow stamens facing upwards. Flowers attract butterflies. Blooms late spring to summer. The hard-shelled fruits are used as snuff boxes. If the fruit are left to dry with the seeds inside they it make amusing rattles for children and are also used as anklets and armlets for dancers to add rhythm when performing. The pulp of the fruit is edible, but is seldom used for that purpose.

Medicinal Uses:

In *African medicine*, the *roots* are used in the *treatment of dysentery* and *bladder complaints*. The *Fried Egg Tree is a native to South Africa.*

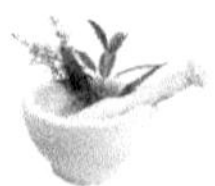

Lesser Swertia

Botanical Name:

Swertia minor

Family:

Gentianaceae (**Gentian family**)

Synonyms:

Ophelia minor, Pleurogyna minor

Common Names:

Lesser Swertia • Kannada: *Kiraatha thiktha* • Marathi: *Lahan chirayat*

Description:

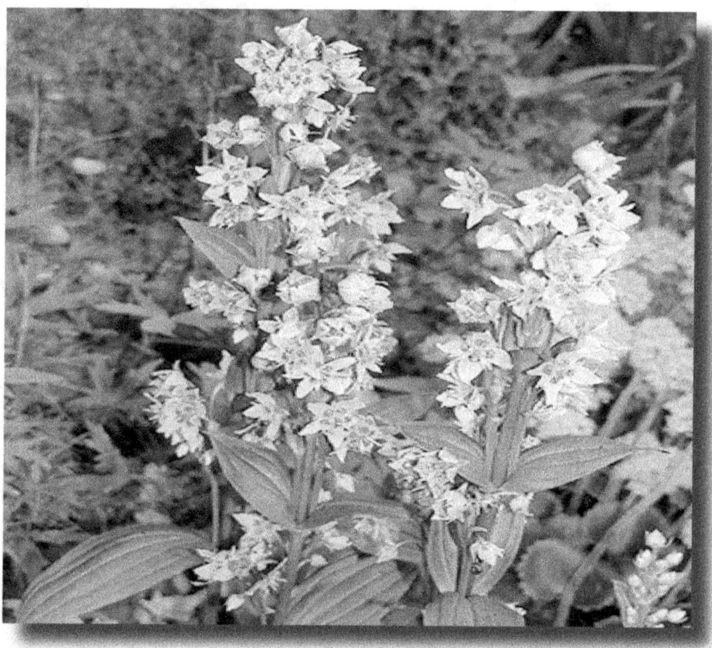

Lesser Swertia is a small annual herb, growing up to 15 cm tall, with 4-winged stem. Stalkless leaves are ovate, 0.5-1 cm long, 5 mm wide, with pointed tip. Flowers are borne in leafy panicle-like cymes. They are 4-or 5-merous, sepal cups divided almost to the base into 4 or 5 ovate sepals, 3-4 mm long, enlarging in fruit. Flowers are 6-7 mm long, with a very short tube, and 4-5 ovate-oblong, pointed petals, with 5 parallel nerves. Each petal has 2 triangular pockets near the base. Stamens are 4-5, with flattened filaments. Lesser Swertia is found in the Western Ghats. Flowering: July-August.

Medicinal Uses:

Leaf decoction is given in *fever*.

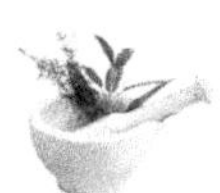

Panicled Swertia

Botanical Name:

Swertia paniculata

Family:

Gentianaceae (**Gentian family**)

Synonyms:

Ophelia paniculata, Ophelia wallichii, Swertia gracilescens

Common Names:

Panicled Swertia • Hindi: *Charaita* • Sanskrit: *Kiratatikta* • Nepali: *Chiraito*

Description:

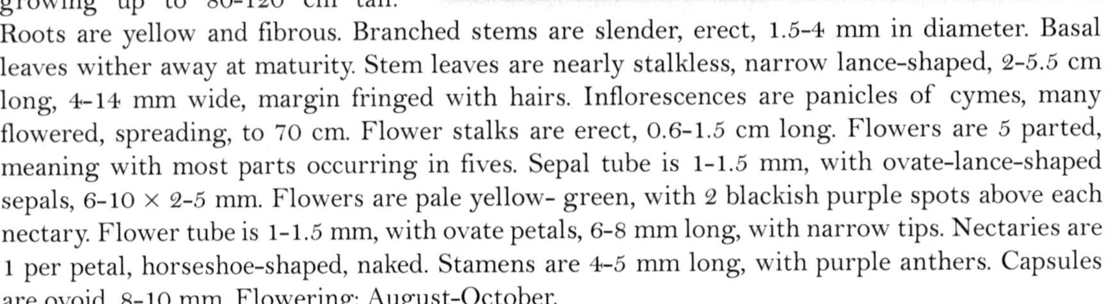

Panicled Swertia is an annual herb, growing up to 80-120 cm tall. Roots are yellow and fibrous. Branched stems are slender, erect, 1.5-4 mm in diameter. Basal leaves wither away at maturity. Stem leaves are nearly stalkless, narrow lance-shaped, 2-5.5 cm long, 4-14 mm wide, margin fringed with hairs. Inflorescences are panicles of cymes, many flowered, spreading, to 70 cm. Flower stalks are erect, 0.6-1.5 cm long. Flowers are 5 parted, meaning with most parts occurring in fives. Sepal tube is 1-1.5 mm, with ovate-lance-shaped sepals, 6-10 × 2-5 mm. Flowers are pale yellow- green, with 2 blackish purple spots above each nectary. Flower tube is 1-1.5 mm, with ovate petals, 6-8 mm long, with narrow tips. Nectaries are 1 per petal, horseshoe-shaped, naked. Stamens are 4-5 mm long, with purple anthers. Capsules are ovoid, 8-10 mm. Flowering: August-October.

Medicinal Uses:

Decoction of the plant is used as a *tonic*. The plant is also used as a *substitute for Chirayita* in the *treatment of malaria* and *other types of fevers.*

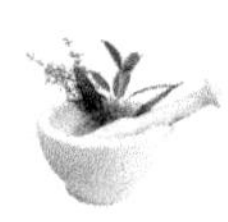

Stone Flower

Botanical Name:
Didymocarpus pedicellatus

Family:
Gesneriaceae (**Gloxinia family**)

Synonyms:
Didymocarpus pedicellata

Common Names:
Stone Flower • Hindi: *Charela, Pattharphori* • Sanskrit: *Shila pushp, Shantapushpi, Pasanbheda* • Nepali: *Kum*

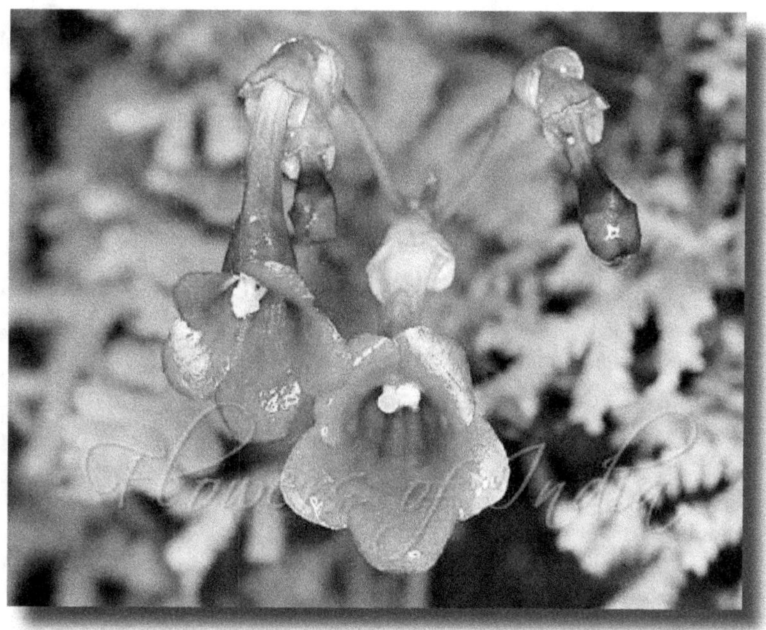

Description:
The Name Stone Flower, and various local Names, probably come from the plant's believed efficacy in curing kidney stones, or probably because it occurs on rocks. It is a usually stemless plant of damp rocks, with 2 large basal leaves with long stalks. Leaves are roundly ovate, rounded toothed. Many reddish purple flowers, 2.5 cm long, occur in clusters, at the end of erect flowering stems, which are about 20 cm tall. Ovate bracts are often fused below. Coloured, rounded sepals form a funnel shaped tube. The flower tube is narrow cylindric with a flaring mouth consisting of 5 rounded petals. Capsule is linear, beaked. Occurs in the Himalayas, from Himachal Pradesh to Arunachal Pradesh, at altitudes of 500-2500 m. Flowering: July-September.

Medicinal Uses:
Stone Flower is a valuable, although a *lesser known medicinal plant*. Traditionally, the Stone Flower is used in the treatment of *renal diseases*, particularly *kidney stones*. According to a hypothesis, the plant is supposed to regulate the *calcium absorption in the body*. The plant is known for its *diuretic effects* and for maintaining *healthy urinary tracts*.

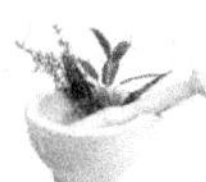

Ceylon Hydrolea

Botanical Name:

Hydrolea zeylanica

Family:

Hydrophyllaceae (**Waterleaf family**)

Synonyms:

Nama zeylanica

Common Names:

Ceylon Hydrolea • Hindi: *Koliary* • Manipuri: *Charang* • Marathi: *Popti, Keriti* • Tamil: *Vellel* • Malayalam: *Cheruvallel* • Bengali: *Isa-langulia, Kasschra* • Konkani: *Kerit*

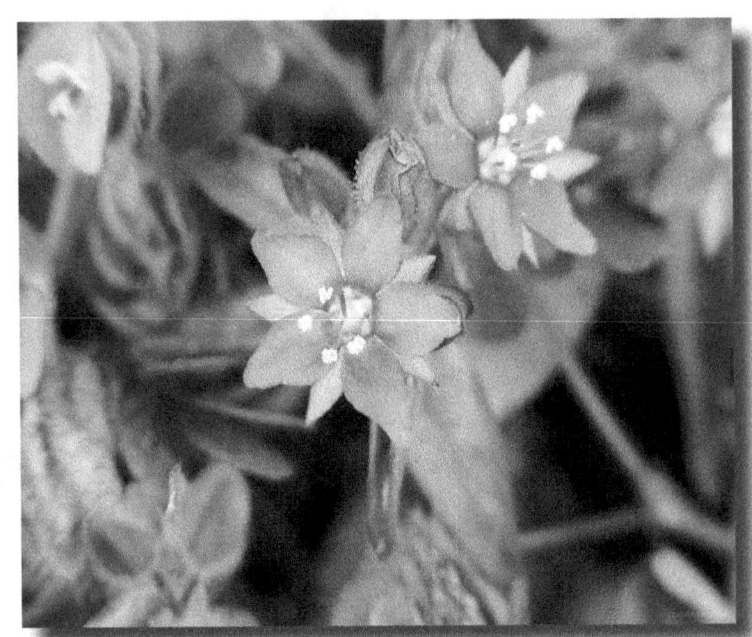

Description:

Ceylon Hydrolea is an annual aquatic herb, ascending or prostrate, sparingly branched, a few cm to 1.2 meters in length, and rooting at the lower nodes. The leaves are lanceolate, 4–10 mm long, and pointed at both ends. The flowers are very numerous, bright blue, and borne in racemes. The sepals are hairy, green, oblong-linear, and about 5 mm long. The flower is 8–10 mm across. The capsule is ovoid, surrounded by the persistent sepals, and contains numerous, minute, oblong seeds. Flowering: October-December.

Medicinal Uses:

The *leaves* are *beaten into pulp and is applied as a poultice.* The leaves are basically considered to have a *cleansing and healing effect* on *neglected and callous ulcers.* They apparently possess some *antiseptic properties.*

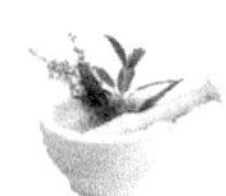

Golden Eye Grass

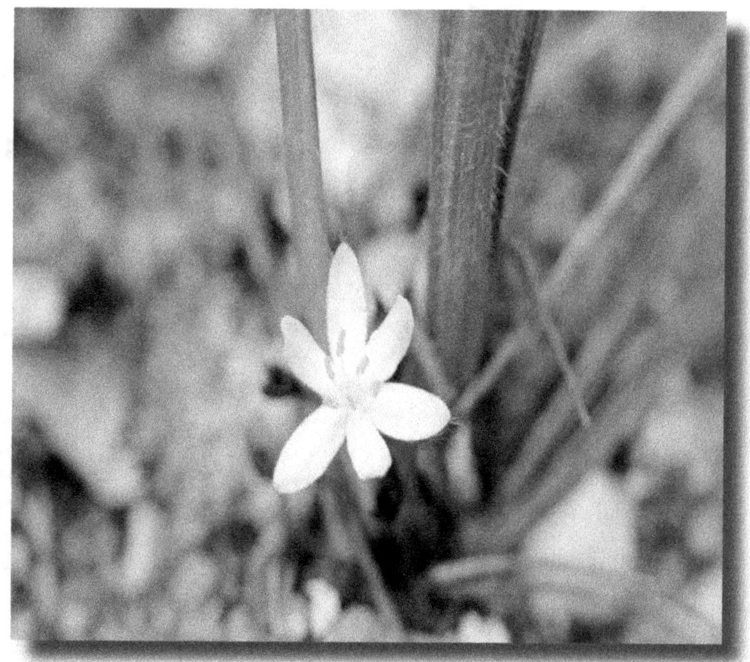

Botanical Name:

Curculigo orchioides

Family:

Hypoxidaceae (**Star Grass family**)

Synonyms:

Curculigo ensifolia, Curculigo brevifolia, Hypoxis orchioides

Common Names:

Golden Eye Grass, Orchid palm grass • Hindi: *Kali musli* • Oriya: *Tala-muli* • Kannada: *Nela tengu* • Malayalam: *Nelppana* • Tamil: *Nilappanaikkilanku* • Bengali: *Talamuli*

Description:

Golden Eye Grass is a herbaceous tuberous perennial with a short or elongate root stock bearing several fleshy lateral roots. The plant can grow up to 10-35 cm tall. Leaves sessile or petiolate 15-45x1.3-2.5 cm, linear or linear lanceolate, tips sometimes rooting, scape very short, clavate. It has hardy leaves and can take shade: the leaves will just get a bit longer in the shade than in full sun shine. During flowering period it open a golden yellow flower at the leaf base every day. This can form a cute miniature plant pot in your room. Flowering: July-August.

Medicinal Uses:

The *rhizomes of the plants* are used for the treatment of *decline in strength, jaundice* and *asthma*. According to *Ayurveda*, the root is heated, aphrodisiac, alternative, appetizer, fattening and useful in the treatment of *piles, biliousness, fatigue, blood related disorders*, etc. According to the *Unani system of medicine*, the root is *carminative, tonic, aphrodisiac, antipyretic* and useful in *bronchitis, ophthalmia, indigestion, vomiting, diarrhoea, lumbago, gonorrhea, gleet, hydrophobia, joint pains*, etc.

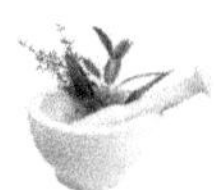

Himalayan Bugle

Botanical Name:
Ajuga lupulina

Family:
Lamiaceae (**Mint family**)

Common Names:
Himalayan Bugle • Nepali: Jhyasuk

Description:
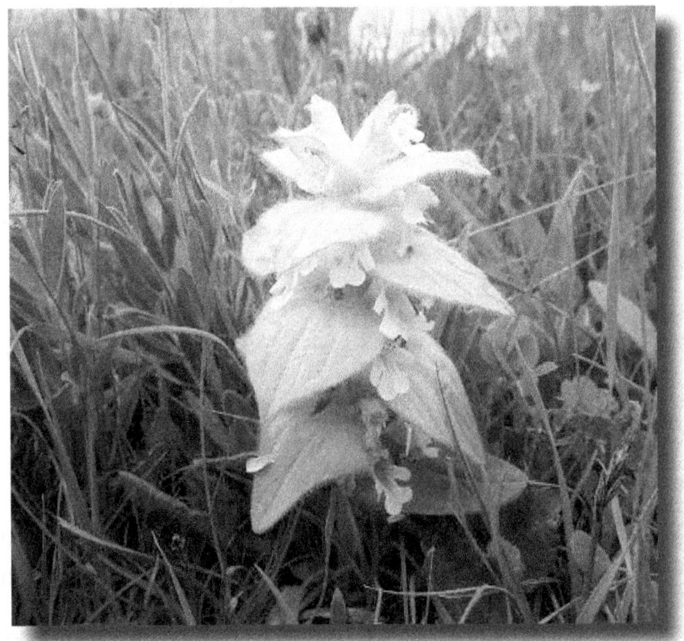

Ajuga or bugle is a genus of about 40-50 species of annual and perennial herbaceous flowering plants in the mint family. Himalayan Bugle is characterized by large densely overlapping, prominently netveined bracts, which almost conceal the flowers. The bracts grow larger and turn red after flowering. Flowers white, whitish green, or whitish yellow with purple lines, narrowly funnelform, 1.8-2.5 cm, sparsely hairy; tube slightly swollen to saccate near base, woolly inside, curved; upper lip straight, 2-lobed, with subcircular lobes; lower lip projected, with middle lobe narrowly flabellate.

Medicinal Uses:
A *decoction of the plant*, *Artemisia sieversiana*, combined with the *Himalayan Bugle* and *Ephedra gerardiana*, is used as *a wash to relieve painful joints*. The *seeds, leaves* and *flowers* of the *Himalayan Bugle* are used in *treating fever, sinusitis, infections, menstrual disorders, swellings, skin diseases* and *paralysis*.

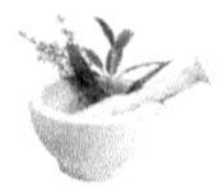

Malabar Catmint

Botanical Name:
Anisomeles malabarica

Family:
Lamiaceae (**Mint family**)

Synonyms:
Anisomeles salviifolia, Nepeta malabarica

Common Names:
Malabar Catmint • Hindi: *Gopoli, Codhara* • Marathi: *Gojibha* • Tamil: *Peyimarutti* • Malayalam: P*erumtumpa, Karintumpa* • Telugu: *Mogabiran, Mogabheri* • Kannada: *Karitumbi, Gandubirana gida* • Oriya: *Vaikuntha* • Konkani: *Kaktumbo* • Sanskrit: *Mahadronah, Vaikunthah*

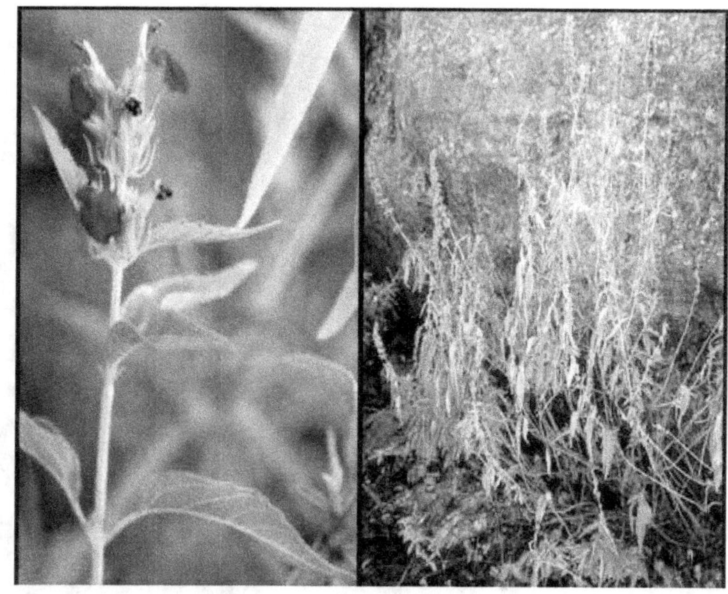

Description:
The Malabar Catmint is a shrubby herb, 0.5-1.5 m tall. Stems are tetragonous, densely villous or woolly. Leaves are ovate to oblong, 3-8 cm x 1.5-3 cm, densely woolly beneath, sparsely hirsute above, hairs 4-celled, petiole 0.5-2.5 cm long, softly woolly. Inflorescence is a single terminal spike, calyx 8.5 mm x 6 mm, longest teeth 3-4 mm long, in fruit 8-10 mm long, teeth hairy inside. Flower up to 1.8 cm long, lower lip about 12 mm x 4 mm, lilac or pale blue, filaments almost at same level, about 8 mm long, style about 1.3 cm long. Nutlets are cylindrical, 1.3 mm x 0.9 mm.

Medicinal Uses:
The whole plant, especially the leaves and the roots are used as an *astringent, carminative, febrifuge* and *tonic.*

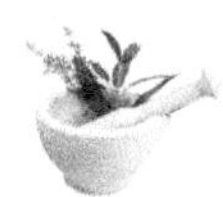

Shady Calamint

Botanical Name:

Clinopodium umbrosum

Family:

Lamiaceae (**Mint family**)

Synonyms:

Calamintha umbrosa, Clinopodium repens, Melissa umbrosum, Satureja umbrosa

Common Names:

Shady Calamint • Hindi: *Birchee* • Nepali: *Suparnasa, Bilajor*

Description:

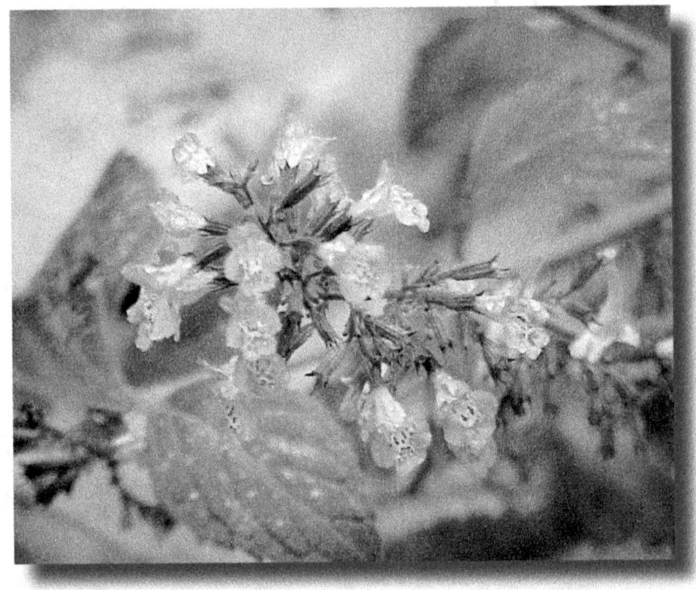

Shady Calamint is a softly hairy perennial herb, found in the Himalayas, from Afghanistan to SE Asia, at altitudes of 1000-3400 m. The plant grows 1-3 ft tall, with short stalked ovate leaves which have sharply toothed margin. Flowers are small, pink or purple, borne in lax few-flowered whorls, with few short slender bracts. Flowers are about 8 mm long, with a sepal tube 6 mm long, with unequal sepals. Sepals have bristly hairs on them. Flowering: April-October.

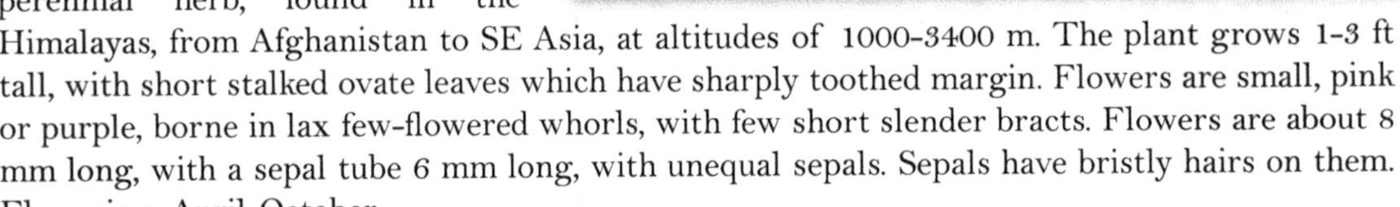

Medicinal Uses:

In *Nepal,* the *juice of the leaves* is applied to *cuts and wounds.*

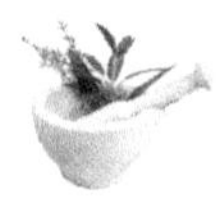

White Dead Nettle

Botanical Name:

Lamium album

Family:

Lamiaceae (**Mint family**)

Common Names:

White Dead Nettle, Blind nettle, Dumb nettle, Deaf nettle, Bee nettle

Description:

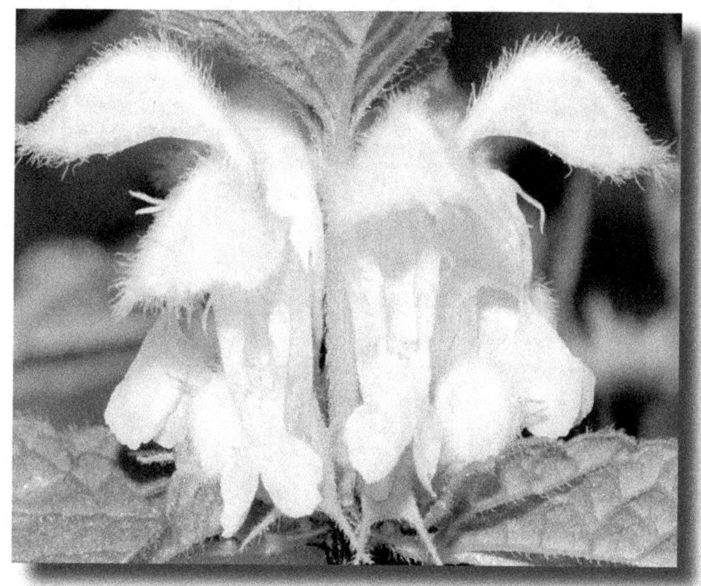

White Deadnettle is a perennial herb found in damp places in Western Himalayas, at altitudes of 1500-3700 m. It grows up to 50-100 cm tall, with green, four-angled stems. Ovate-heart-shaped leaves are 2.5-8 cm long and 2-5 cm broad, with coarsely toothed margin. The leaves appear superficially similar to those of the Stinging nettle Urtica dioica but do not sting, hence the common Name "dead nettle". Lower leaves have stalks while the upper ones are stalk-less. The flowers are white, produced in a few whorls, vertically separated, on the upper part of the stem. The flowers whorls arise from the axils of the upper oppositely arranged leaves. The flowers are 1.5-2.5 cm long, 2-lipped, with a curved flower-tube with a swollen base. The upper lip is hooded over the stamens, and is quite hairy, with white hairs forming a fringe on the hood. The lower lip smaller, bilobed. The young leaves are edible, and can be used in salads or cooked as a vegetable. The plant also has a number of uses in herbal medicine. Bees are attracted to the flowers which contain nectar or pollen, hence the plant is sometimes called the Bee Nettle. Flowering: April-July.

Medicinal Uses:

The White Dead Nettle is an *astringent* and *demulcent herb* that is chiefly used as a *uterine tonic*, to arrest *intermenstrual bleeding* and to reduce *excessive menstrual flow*. It is a *traditional treatment* for *abnormal vaginal discharge* and is sometimes taken to *relieve painful periods.*

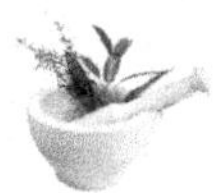